THE ULTIMATE TRAIL running HANDBOOK

GET FIT, CONFIDENT AND SKILLED-UP TO GO FROM 5K TO 50K

CLAIRE MAXTED

BLOOMSBURY SPORT
LONDON · OXFORD · NEW YORK · NEW DELHI · SYDNEY

BLOOMSBURY SPORT
Bloomsbury Publishing Plc
50 Bedford Square, London, WC1B 3DP, UK
29 Earlsfort Terrace, Dublin 2, Ireland

BLOOMSBURY, BLOOMSBURY SPORT and the Diana logo are trademarks
of Bloomsbury Publishing Plc

ISBN: PB: 978-1-4729-7484-6; eBook: 978-1-4729-7483-9

6 8 10 9 7 5

Typeset in Verlag by Lee-May Lim
Printed and bound in China by Toppan Leefung Printing

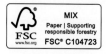

To find out more about our authors and books visit www.bloomsbury.com
and sign up for our newsletters

CONTENTS

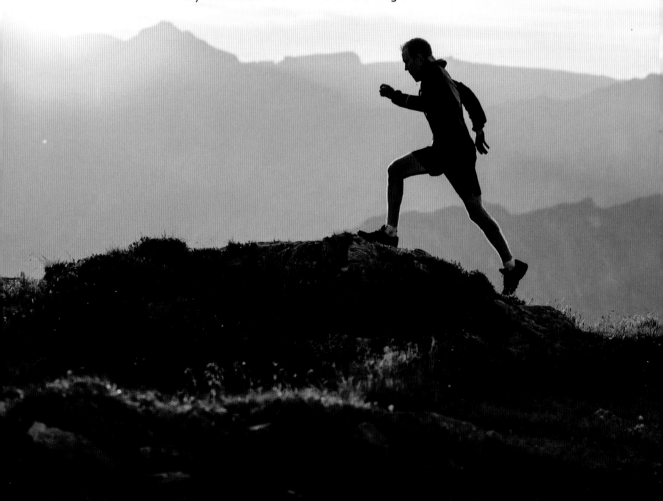

TRAIL RUNS AREN'T JUST ABOUT THE POWER IN YOUR LEGS,
THEY ALSO REVEAL THE SIZE OF YOUR HEART
AND THE STRENGTH OF YOUR MIND.

TRAIL RUNNING HELPS ORDINARY PEOPLE
DO EXTRAORDINARY THINGS

KEEP RUNNING OFF-ROAD
KEEP BUILDING A BETTER YOU

By Alistair Jones @RunningMrJones

FOREWORD

Claire Maxted is ace. I've got a lot to thank her for. And, seeing as you've got this book in your hands, so do you. We'll get onto you in a moment. But if you wouldn't mind, let's start with me...

I first met Claire in the Lake District – I'd just completed my first ever trail race and she was on the other side of a camera asking me about it. Fair to say, even at that early stage, the trails had me smitten.

I arrived in Keswick fresh from a lengthy quest to break three hours in a road marathon. There's certainly pleasure and satisfaction to be gleaned training for and achieving a longstanding goal like that. But after many years with my head buried in a Garmin, suddenly I found myself cresting a magnificent fell on a glorious spring morning, the sublime radiance of the Lake District unfolding below me, soft earth underfoot, thighs burning, nostrils gasping fresh, unpolluted air... and I was blissfully unaware of trivialities like time and pace. Quite simply, in that moment, there was nowhere I'd rather be, nothing I'd rather be doing.

When she interviewed me afterwards, Claire sensed my nascent enthusiasm and over the next few months set about helping to mould, direct and strengthen it. Soon I was gleefully spending weekends running in the Surrey Hills, Dorset Downs or Brecon Beacons, anywhere there was nature crying out to be explored. I started signing up for fell races, trail marathons, a 100-mile run along the length of the South Downs

Way, even the notorious Berghaus Dragon's Back Race, a multi-day mountain ultra over every peak in Wales. I loved every lung-busting second.

These days, whenever I see a big hill, I have a strange yearning to run up it. That's partly Claire's fault. Like I say I have lots to thank her for.

So, where does all of this leave you? It leaves you about to embark on the most magnificent journey you could possibly imagine. Trail running is a wonderful sport, as welcoming and inclusive as it is spectacular.

It's going to leave you sweaty and muddy and a little smelly. It's going to leave you with wet trainers, new friends and a bucket load of unforgettable experiences. It's going to leave you fitter than you've ever been.

It's going to leave you cresting a magnificent fell on a glorious spring morning, the sublime radiance of the Lake District unfolding below you, soft earth underfoot, thighs burning, nostrils gasping fresh, unpolluted air...

There is no more authentic trail running messenger than Claire. So take her tips, appreciate her advice.

And get stuck in!

Vassos Alexander
Radio Sports Reporter

I remember the first time I met Claire, it was during the first edition of The Salomon Glen Coe Skyline, and her happiness for trail running was shining so bright. It's always fun to do interviews, but even more with someone who is really passionate and has a lot of knowledge about the subject. And that I can tell you, Claire is and has!

I can't remember now whether Claire was running the race or if she was just all over the course following the runners, but from many of the races I've done, she is there to report and to write about either the race, specific runners, topics, destination, etc.

From reading her book I can see how so much knowledge and happiness transmits through her writing – if you are in the slightest bit interested in trail running this book is for you!

It has a bit of everything. Like the exercises that can be very good for all the small muscles trail runners need to use for maximum strength. It also has good recovery tips, tips on nutrition, races, training and everything in-between. The content lives up to the name, that is for sure.

Even though I might be considered an experienced trail runner, I still enjoyed this book. I think if you like the subject it's always interesting to read about it and you might find new ways, to look at things, new thoughts and inspiration.

Hope to see you on the trails!

Emelie Forsberg
Record-breaking trail and ultra runner

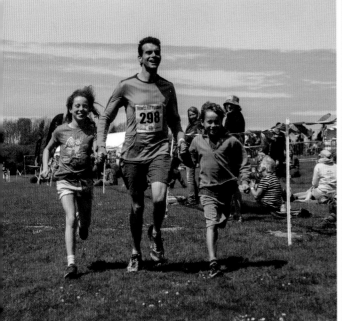

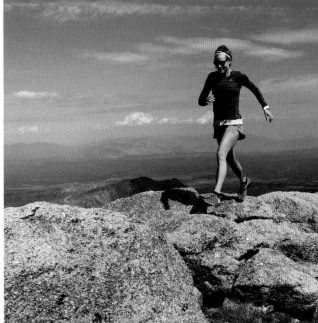

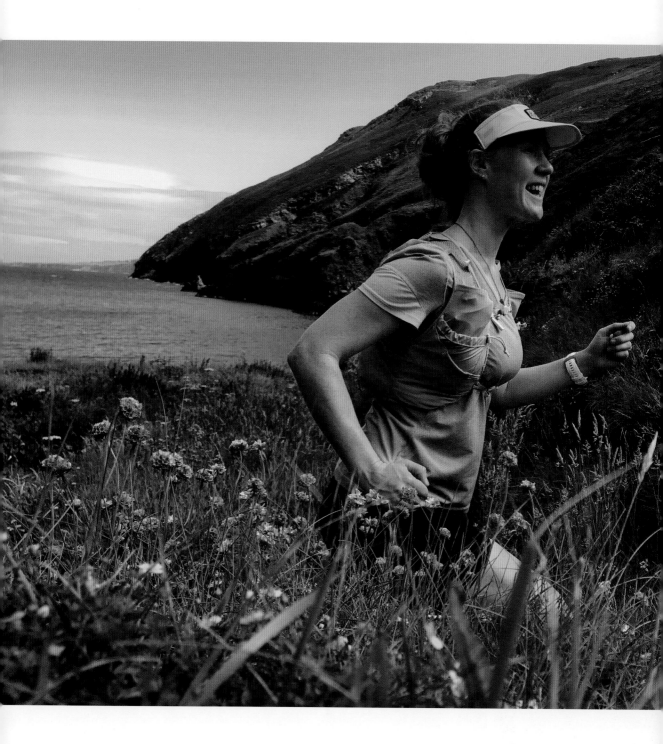

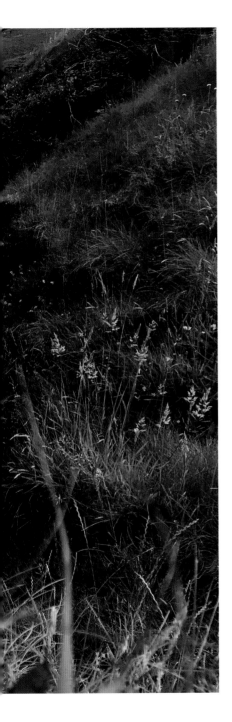

WELCOME

Congratulations for picking up this book, whether you're just starting out on your trail running journey or looking to hone your skills with the expert tips, you are in for an exciting adventure off-road.

MY STORY – I HATED RUNNING!

I hated running at school. I lived in fear of the beep test, sports day, House cross country and even worse, the communal showers afterwards. Running was always fast, competitive and therefore horrible. Luckily, I got involved with hiking at school instead and loved the steadier pace, mountain views and adventure. At uni, I decided to cure my running phobia because I was getting a beer gut! I forced myself to do it, soon veering off-road into parks and woods to find more interesting routes. I knew about this terrifying thing super-fit people did called fell running, so one winter I borrowed a very badly fitting bumbag and huffed and puffed (mainly walked) my way up a tiny Lake District hill, then slipped over on the frosty descent. It wasn't until I was working on *Trail* (the walking magazine) that I discovered the Lakeland Trails beginner-friendly trail running events – 10ish miles (16km) on beautiful hilly courses in the Lake District. I loved it! It was hiking slightly sped up, and the downhills were tremendous fun. So it was with great pleasure that I co-founded *Trail Running* magazine and edited it until 2017. Now I run Wild Ginger Running, the trail and ultra running advice and inspiration channel on YouTube. This wonderful sport gives you double the adventure and triple the accomplishment in a fun and friendly community full of fantastic, like-minded people. All you need is a pair of grippy trainers and a sense of adventure. And the best thing? It's brilliant fun, both mentally and physically. Enjoy your own journey into trail running.

Happy trails,

Claire Maxted

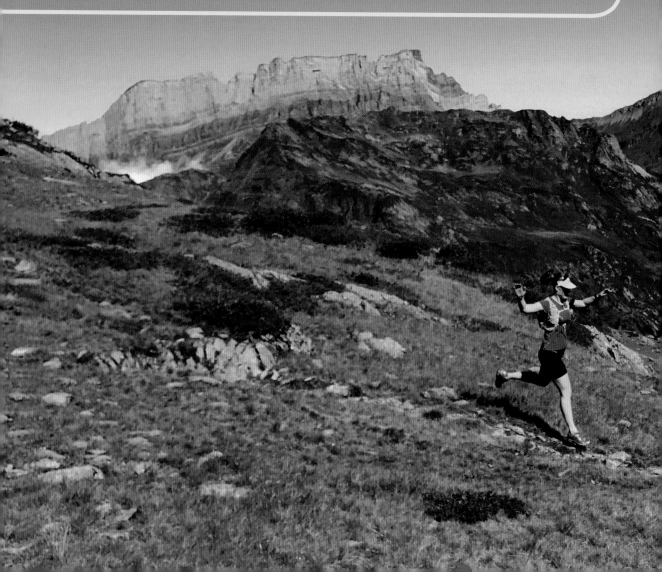

1

QUICK START

Later chapters will cover the aspects mentioned here in more detail, but if you're positively raring to get trail running, this chapter will give you the info you need to get off to a quick start.

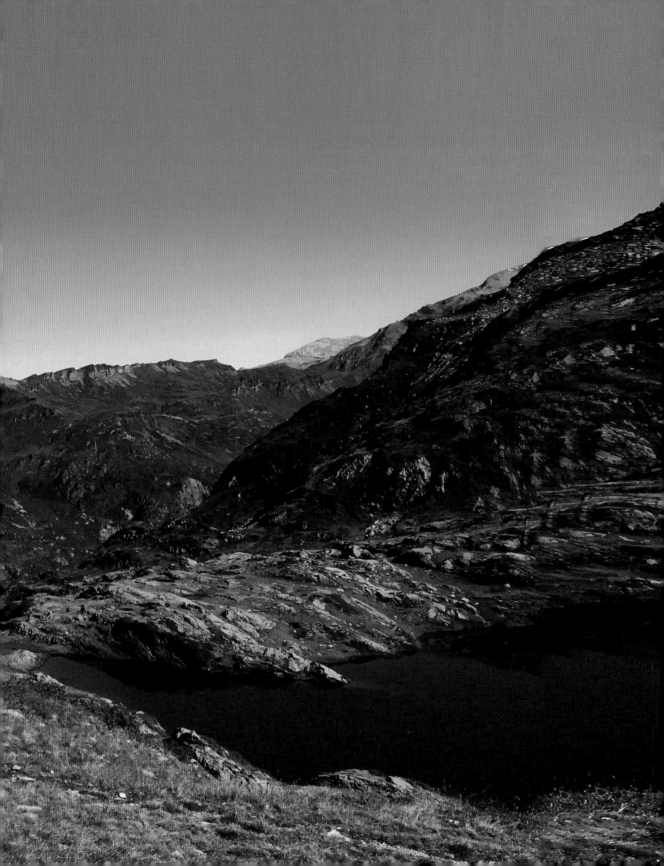

WHAT IS TRAIL RUNNING?

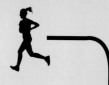

Trail running bridges the gap between easily accessible road running and skilful fell running over pathless mountains. Trail running is mainly on clear paths and bridleways, over hills, around mountains and lakes, and along coastlines, disused railway tracks and canal towpaths. Basically, whenever your feet aren't hitting tarmac but there's a nice path that isn't along an alarming rocky knife-edge ridge, that's trail running.

ROAD RUNNING

Running on pavements next to roads, dodging people armed with umbrellas and buggies, stopping at traffic lights, breathing in fumes. Unless you're in a race where they've closed the roads and you can run wherever you like, whoo! Still doesn't make up for the fact that it's a road...

TRAIL RUNNING

Running on clear trails on paths, bridleways and tracks, both urban and rural, as long as there's no tarmac. Trails might take you beside canals and rivers, through forests and fields, over stiles and up hills and mountains with a soundtrack of breeze and birdsong – freedom, exploration and adventure await!

HASHING

A super-fun social, hare and hounds-style run for all abilities, where the leaders lay a flour trail for the rest to follow, with false trails for the faster ones to discover and feed back to the rest of the group so the slower ones run the right way. Often on trails and almost always followed by a pub, what's not to like?

> *'Nothing beats the glow you get post trail running. You don't need an expensive gym pass; a pair of trainers and sense of adventure opens a whole new world.'*
>
> Matt Swaine, former Trail magazine editor, co-founder of Trail Running magazine

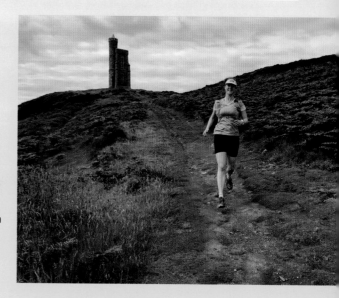

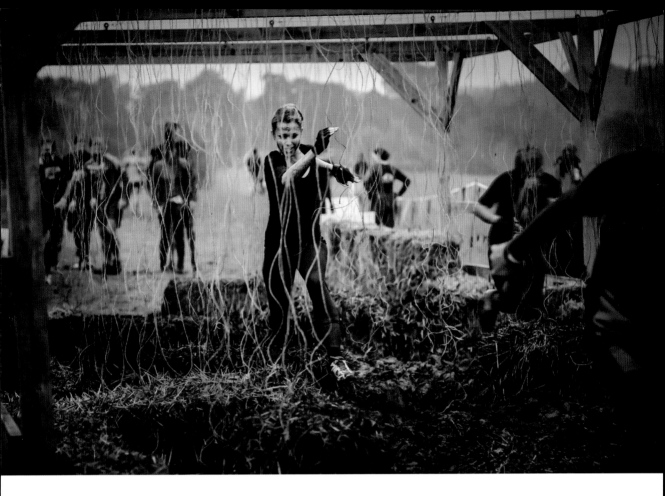

CROSS COUNTRY (XC)

Kind of the old-school version of trail running, but with more of a short, competitive, 'let's blast round this muddy park' vibe than today's trail running. This is the sport I used to live in fear of at school!

OBSTACLE COURSE RACING (OCR)

Based on the famous winter Tough Guy races from the 1990s, with freezing water plunges, army assault course obstacles, barbed wire crawls and dangling electric shock wires. The latter two are rare now, but everything else has got bigger, including huge water jumps, monkey bars, hay bale mountains and slippery walls.

ULTRA RUNNING

Running a flabbergastingly long way has become extremely popular over the last few years. The definition of ultra is simply any race that is more than the marathon distance of 26.2 miles (42.2km). Popular distances are 50km (31 miles), 50 miles (80km), 100km (62 miles) and the much-coveted 100 miles (160km). There are even longer multi-day races too.

FELL RUNNING

The most hardcore kind of running – think tiny shorts, club vests and racing up high hills and mountains, navigating the quickest way possible over rough, pathless ground. Fell runners welcome newcomers, but the sensible will ease themselves in gradually with trail running and hiking first. Also called hill running in Scotland.

ORIENTEERING

A thrilling combination of fitness, navigation skills and strategy, often rural but also urban events. You get a map with either a linear route with checkpoints (controls) to find as quickly as possible, or a score course where you collect as many controls as possible in a given time, losing points if you're late back.

MOUNTAIN MARATHONS

The ultimate test of navigation and mountain survival skills. Pairs complete linear or score-orienteering courses in harsh, remote and pathless mountainside, carrying all the kit and food they need for two days. Pick the right partner as spooning in the tiniest, lightest tent possible is mandatory at mid-camp.

MOUNTAIN RUNNING

A discipline with a global governing body called the World Mountain Running Association (WMRA), holding world championships on off-road, mountainous terrain but with clearly marked courses that avoid dangerous sections.

SKYRUNNING

Very popular in Europe, Skyrunning favours mountain fitness over navigation with waymarked courses over testing, technical terrain at high altitude. In the UK, what we lack in altitude we make up for in rocky, knife-edge ridges and scrambling.

HILL WALKING

Hill and mountain walking is a fantastic intro to trail and fell running as it gives you a whole raft of transferable skills – endurance, navigation, mountain skills and moving over technical ground. Speed walking is an essential skill for off-road runners too.

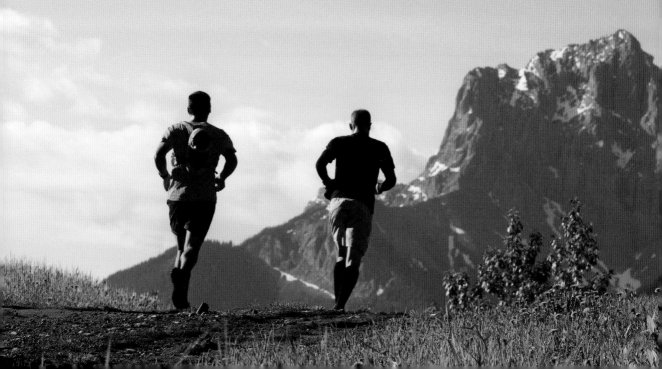

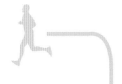

TRAIL VS ROAD

Obviously I'm biased, but trail running is 100 gazillion per cent more exciting than road running! If there were a pill containing all the physical and mental health benefits trail running gives you it would be worth millions. Clever clogs all over the world agree that exercise in nature is one of the best gifts you can give your mind and body.

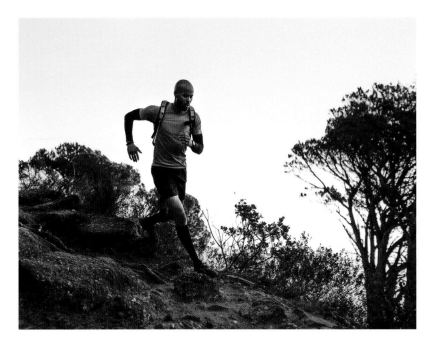

'Why do I love trail running? No stopwatch, no set distance, no agenda. Just you and the countryside — superb.'

Paul Larkins, Trail Running *magazine editor*

1 Trail running is way more fun! You get to explore the paths and fields around your local area or further afield, discovering views, monuments, trees and lakes you never knew existed before! There's no stopping at traffic lights, looking around for cars, less people to dodge round – it's pure freedom and a time to play.

2 Spending time in nature can massively boost your mental health, so while road running keeps your body fit, trail running is a health pill for your brain. Running through beautiful landscapes, listening to the birds and breathing in the fresh air reduces your stress levels and makes you feel better about life and the world in general. You're guaranteed to come back smiling and refreshed.

3 Breathing deeply on city streets isn't as healthy for you as running in the fresh countryside and mountain air, where the pollution levels are exponentially lower. Step away from the exhaust fumes of cars, vans and lorries barrelling past, and fill your lungs with the clean country breeze.

4 Your legs will thank you for taking them away from the repetitive pavement pounding. Trail running uses different muscles every single time you put your foot down on the ground because it's always different underfoot; rocky, grassy, muddy – you name it, it's always a new way to land. You'll also use more of your core and upper body to stabilise yourself – and more energy burned equals more cake, right?

5 Running into the unknown gives you the opportunity to learn new skills, whether that's getting your brain around tackling rocky downhills to absorbing basic map-reading knowledge as you explore. Start to plan routes around your local area, then take your adventures to National Parks as you pick up the skills you need to navigate yourself safely through even more interesting countryside.

'Running 15 minutes a day protects you from heart attacks and strokes.'

The American Journal of Medicine

Running for 30 minutes 5 times a week strengthens your lungs and diaphragm for deeper, more effective breathing.'

American Lung Association

Running for 2.5 hours per week helps prevent bone-weakening conditions like osteoporosis.'

NHS

'Running helps you lose more weight more quickly than walking.'

Medicine & Science in Sports & Exercise journal

'Running reduces the risk of 13 different types of cancer.'

Cancer Research UK

'Running in green spaces increases energy, positivity, satisfaction and motivation and decreases tension, confusion, anger and depression.'

Peninsula College of Medicine and Dentistry

'25 minutes' running in a green space reduces fatigue and enhances brain power and creativity.'

British Journal of Sports Medicine

'Running helps you get the recommended 7–9 hours of sleep and helps with insomnia.'

Advances in Preventive Medicine journal

RUNNING SAVED MY LIFE

'I came to running late in life, at a time when mental health wasn't the openly discussed topic it thankfully is now. Trail running is the ultimate release for me. I can allow myself time not to think, be anxious or relentlessly negative. I just clear my mind and take in the beauty of it all – even in torrential downpours, or clambering up a muddy hill – the surroundings soak up that awful energy I've been carrying around. All that self-doubt and overthinking. Worries melt away. Road running is great, but trail running is completely different and it has saved me from being under a cloud on so many occasions. I feel so lucky to have it in my life.'

SCOTT BARTLETT, LONDON

TRAIL RUNNING MYTHS

Sometimes sharing a trail running fear or problem on social media can bring up a whole host of different answers – not all of them based on scientific fact. So here are the key trail running myths busted.

MYTH:
You must buy the latest running shoe

BUSTED:
There can be a lot of hype over the latest new trail running shoe. Maybe it's the barefoot craze, a reviewer waxing lyrical or one from a popular brand that all the top athletes are wearing. But the best shoe for you is the one that feels most comfy for miles and miles. So try on as many as you can in the shop, run around in them if they let you (a good shop will have a way of allowing you to do this), and go with the one that suits you, not everyone else.

MYTH:
Trail running is only possible in hills and mountains

BUSTED:
Trail running covers a whole variety of landscapes because all it means is that you're avoiding pavements and roads to run instead on paths, tracks and bridleways, which can be found in both urban and rural areas.

MYTH:
You must run up all the hills

BUSTED:
Definitely not. If you go to any big race, even the top runners will power hike (a fancy name for walking fast) up particularly steep or long hills. The longer the race and the steeper the climb, the more likely walking will be more efficient.

MYTH:
Runners have to be tall, long-limbed and lean

BUSTED:
Runners can be whatever shape and size they were made. If you run, you are a runner, and that is a scientific fact.

MYTH:
Running is bad for your knees

BUSTED:
Potentially, you can have knee problems as a runner, which you can strengthen, rehab or aid using poles (see p. 165), but mostly running is good for your bones and joints, helping to prevent bone-weakening conditions such as osteoporosis and strengthening the muscles around the knees.

MYTH:
You must overstuff yourself with pasta before a race

BUSTED:
No. As long as you haven't completely starved yourself and overtrained before a big race, and eaten healthily until you are satisfied, your body will have fully stocked your muscles with as much energy as they can hold so they'll be raring to go on race day.

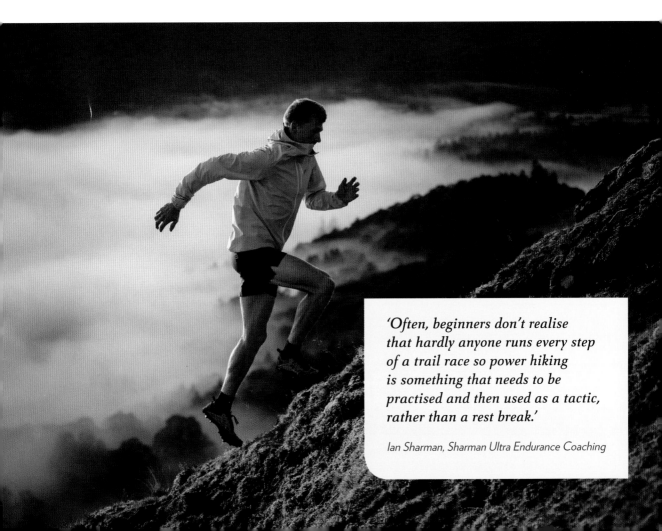

'Often, beginners don't realise that hardly anyone runs every step of a trail race so power hiking is something that needs to be practised and then used as a tactic, rather than a rest break.'

Ian Sharman, Sharman Ultra Endurance Coaching

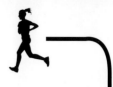

WHERE ARE THE TRAILS?

Great news. You don't have to live in obviously picturesque areas such as the Peak District or Cornwall to find beautiful running routes through green fields, forests and along rivers. Even if you live in the middle of a huge, busy city like Birmingham, I can guarantee you're not more than a few miles from an exciting trail. You just have to know where to look and who to ask.

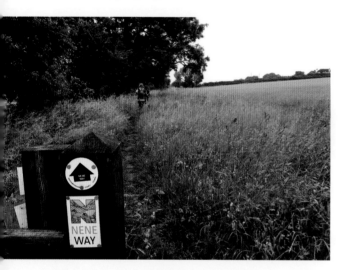

START EXPLORING

Basically, the moment you turn off the pavements and leave the roads behind, that's trail running, so there may be many more local trails than you thought. For example, your local park counts. Is there a canal towpath near you? Or woodland, fields and meadows? Have you seen a footpath or bridleway sign on the way to the shops or commuting to work? If the answer to any of these is 'yes' then grab your running pack (see pp. 144–145 for safety and what to take) and start exploring those areas.

TALK TO OTHERS

If you're in a local running club, Facebook group or online gathering, ask about local trails. I know people who've lived in my town for 20 years and never knew about this amazing former quarry full of trails on the outskirts because they never explored or asked anyone. I found it by ducking through a gap in a hedge that had been intriguing me. The feeling of discovering a new trail is uplifting.

LOOK ON RUNNING APPS

See where others are running on apps such as MapMyRun and Strava. If they run into areas with no roads or through green bits, copy them and have your own adventure. Chat with them in the comments – they might know about even more trails for you to explore.

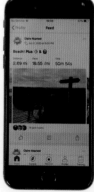

LOOK AT RACE ROUTES

If there are trail races locally, look at their routes on the organiser's website and see if you can find your way round. Just make sure the organiser hasn't had to gain special permission from a landowner to run through certain areas – outside of a race event, you must stick to rights of way and permitted paths (*see* p. 53). Better still, do the race! If it's waymarked then signage, other runners or marshals will guide you round.

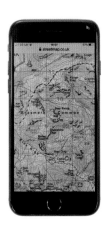

VLOGS AND BLOGS

Google trail runs in your area and see if bloggers or YouTubers have covered any routes near you. When I make Wild Ginger Running YouTube films of trail running routes I sometimes put a map at the end so you can see exactly where I've been.

LOOK AT A MAP

Get your local Ordnance Survey (OS) map 1:25,000 scale or look at OS maps online for free through Bing Maps or Streetmap. Zoom to 1:25,000 scale, find your road and familiarise yourself with the roads you usually run on. Then branch out to follow the footpaths and bridleways – green dotted and dashed lines. These are rights of way and you can run on them. Turn to pp. 56–57 for more map-reading info – it's easier than you might think.

MY STORY

TRAILS ARE EVERYWHERE!

'I started road running in 2018 and then started to watch YouTube videos about running. There, I found trail running and thought it looked amazing – runners in great mountains all around the world. I then thought: "Wow! I need to find some hills and mountains to run up." I kept driving to the mountains until I found a heat map on the app of my new Suunto running watch. It showed loads of trails in my local area – who knew you could run over farmland on paths and bridleways? I was very happy as I could suddenly run on trails less than a mile from my house! I've now found even more using an OS map, double win!'

GUY GREATOREX, CHESHIRE

TRAIL HACK

AVOID GETTING LOST

When you're exploring new trails, keep looking back to familiarise yourself with the views you should be expecting on the return journey. Church spires, tall buildings and communication towers are useful directional aids. Then, when you turn round, it's easier to retrace your steps. Take photos on your phone and make stone or stick arrows beside the path to jog your memory too.

ESSENTIAL GEAR

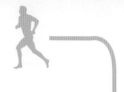

The great thing about trail running is that you don't need a ton of kit. Here are the bare essentials, which you might already have in your wardrobe, especially if you're a road runner. Buy from independent running shops whenever you can; their well-trained staff will help you make the right choice.

RUNNING SHOES

Road trainers or trail shoes, whatever you usually run in, will be fine on easy trails to start with. If you've never run before, try on as many pairs as you can in a shop, wearing your running socks. Jog about and choose the pair that fit the best and feel most comfortable with a similar heel-to-toe drop (height difference between the heel and the toe, *see p. 134*) to the shoes you spend most time in; this will help avoid lower leg injury.

SOCKS

Sports socks are heavenly with their comfort pads, air-venting channels and anti-slip elastication but this is also reflected in the price, so if you don't already own a sports pair, use your normal socks to start with and upgrade as time and cash flow allows.

SPORTS BRA

An absolute essential, especially for those with medium- to large-sized boobs. Beat painful bounce and irreversible strain on your Cooper's ligaments (the ones that help support the breasts; if these stretch, your breasts sag) with a well-fitting sports bra designed for maximum impact.

TOP AND BOTTOMS

A technical, sweat-wicking (gets rid of moisture quickly) T-shirt or long-sleeved top is best, but use any top you feel comfortable in for your first runs. Stretchy shorts and leggings rather than heavy jogging bottoms are easier to run in, and won't drag if the ankle area gets wet.

JACKET

A light wind- or waterproof sports jacket is handy to start running in, then you can tie it round your waist as you warm up. It's best to take a light extra layer of some kind for most runs just in case you need to stop, walk or help someone else.

WATCH

There's no need for an all-singing, all-dancing GPS watch straight away; your phone or a simple watch is all you need to finish your run on time and work out your rough average pace.

SUNNIES

Ones that don't slip off your soon-to-be-sweaty nose are vital, so test yours for slippage and invest in a pair with rubber nose and arm grips if you find them falling down. If you wear a cap or visor, you may not need sunglasses.

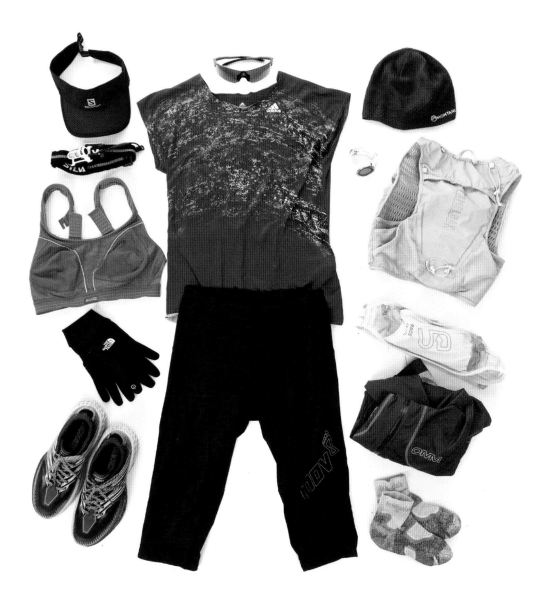

HAT, CAPS AND GLOVES

If it's cold, a headband or hat and gloves are a necessity, and for hot weather, a headband, visor or cap that can be dipped in a river help to cool you down.

HEAD TORCH

For running in the dark you'll need a light head torch with 200–300 lumens of brightness to see enough of the trail.

RUNNING PACK OR BUMBAG

If you want to run further or in colder weather, it's worth investing in a 5-litre running pack or 3-litre bumbag to carry water, phone, keys, a snack and an extra layer.

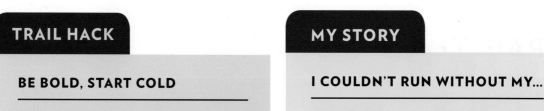

TRAIL HACK

BE BOLD, START COLD

Start running with one less layer than feels comfortable – after 10 minutes of warming up or steady jogging you'll be warm. Carry an extra layer in your pack or round your waist in case you have to stop or slow down.

MY STORY

I COULDN'T RUN WITHOUT MY...

'I couldn't go for a run without my GPS watch. If you go for a run in the forest and there isn't a watch to record it, did it really happen? [Some might disagree with this sentiment!] I can't actually imagine running without one these days. I train using a combination of heart rate and pace and my watch can be set with upper and lower limits to alert you if you go too fast/slow or your heart rate gets too high/low. It's brilliant to avoid overtraining as you build up to higher mileage.'

AMES BASSETT, ISLE OF MAN

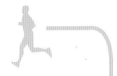

TRAIL TECHNIQUE

The biggest difference between trails and roads is the fact that they're a good deal lumpier. There are more unexpected obstacles, swift directional changes and testing gradients on paths and footpaths, so here's a quick guide to the technique you need to tackle them.

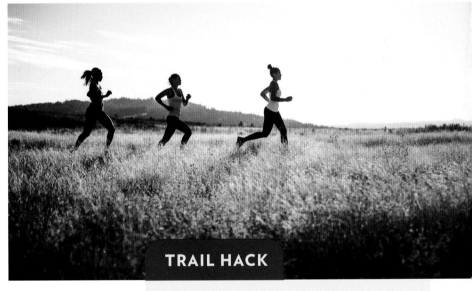

'Off-road running is fun! It's playful, like dancing.'

Kilian Jornet,
Team Salomon

UNEVEN TERRAIN

It's tempting to look down at your feet the whole time once the land gets lumpy, but try to keep scanning the trail from your feet to 2–5m (6.5–16.5ft) ahead. That way, your brain will have more time to process the info on the upcoming route and pass it to your feet.

PICK A LINE

When faced with a rockier or muddier section, look ahead for the easiest way across. This might involve hopping from one rock to another, or looking for flat sections or patches of vegetation that might be grippier. A good way to improve on this if you're running with others is to watch where more experienced trail runners put their feet and follow their lead.

TRAIL HACK

RUN SLOWER

Many runners (especially beginners) fixate on speed, but for trail running it pays to slow down and pace yourself, especially at the start of a route or race, negotiating the terrain steadily and efficiently and saving energy for testing terrain and hills ahead.

UPHILLS

Enjoy the challenge! Lean slightly forwards from the ankles rather than waist, drive from the hips, extend the leg out behind you, take smaller steps and drive with the arms. Go slower so your breathing rate doesn't get too high, easing into a comfortable rhythm and pacing yourself. Break down longer hills by aiming for certain trees or rocks along the way.

DOWNHILLS

Time to fly! Have your arms out wider for balance, think like a ballet dancer and look a few more metres ahead as you nip quickly from foot to foot, not putting too much trust in any foot placement in case the ground shifts, always looking for the next rock or patch of ground on which to place your foot. Go slowly to start with and practise on forgiving grassy slopes.

TOP THREE ANKLE-STRENGTH MOVES

Trail running requires your ankles to be strong and supple, so do any of these exercises in spare moments, for example waiting for the kettle to boil:

1. Calf raises: 3 x 15 repetitions.
2. Stand on one leg for 30–60 seconds, then the other x 5.
3. Single-leg squats: 3 x 15 repetitions each side.

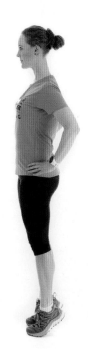
1.

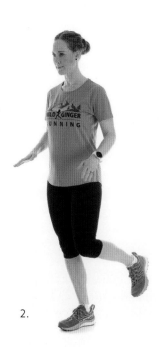
2.

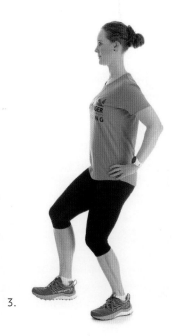
3.

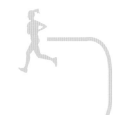

EAT RIGHT

Trail running is more of a whole-body workout that burns more energy than road running as all sorts of muscles are engaged to stabilise yourself on rough terrain. It's a great way to balance out treats such as cake, pies and beer, but of course you'll want to mainly follow your usual healthy diet full of different-coloured vegetables, lean meats, fruits and slow-release carbs for the best performance. Tasty, healthy recipes are covered in chapter 6, but these simple guidelines will keep you on the right track.

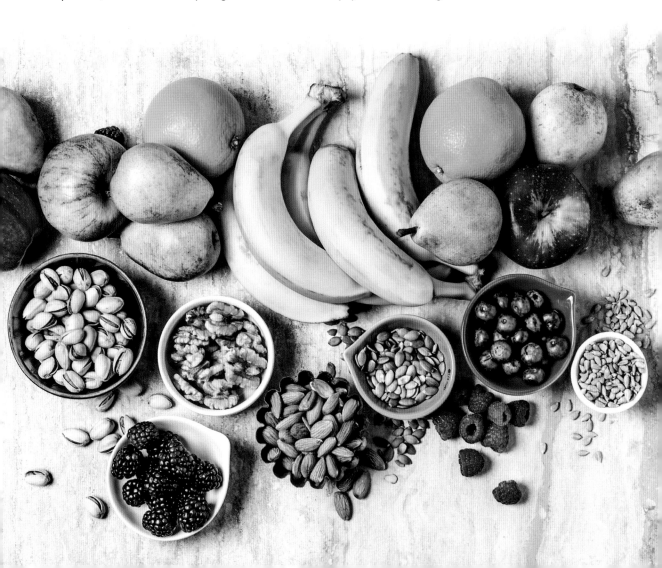

1 ENJOY YOUR GREENS

Eat plenty of leafy green vegetables and different-coloured vegetables for the best possible spread of nutrients and minerals – vital for the best training, performance and a quick recovery.

2 EAT A GOOD BALANCE

The British Nutrition Foundation recommend eating at least five portions of fruit and veg a day, wholegrain and high-fibre carbohydrates, two portions of sustainably sourced fish (one oily), more beans and pulses and less red and processed meat, unsaturated oils, and low-fat, low-sugar dairy and alternative products.

3 AVOID HIGH-SUGAR AND PROCESSED FOODS

As a runner, avoid high-sugar foods unless you're using them to fuel long runs or workouts more than 60–90 minutes long. Making food from scratch is best to avoid extra sugar, salt, fat and strange additives in processed food. Batch cook meals, freeze them in airtight boxes, then defrost and reheat as required so you can eat nutritious home-cooked food on busy evenings.

4 EAT HEALTHY SNACKS

If you eat enough in three regular meals a day, then you reduce the need to snack, which saves time, brain power and also your teeth. However, if you do feel hungry between meals try healthier snacks such as fruit, dried fruit and nuts, carrot and cucumber sticks or rice cakes with peanut butter.

TRAIL HACK

NO GUILT REQUIRED!

Rather than seeing foods as good or bad, or not-guilty versus guilty, try thinking of foods in terms of the nutritional value they bring into your body. Look at the ingredients and the nutritional breakdown of foods to learn more about them. Focus on eating wholesome food rather than trying to stop yourself eating processed sugary, fatty foods.

TOP 10 FOODS TO FUEL YOUR LONG RUN

When running for longer than 60–90 minutes you might need a snack, washed down with a drink. You don't need to fork out for expensive energy bars – here are some great, easy, low-cost fuel sources to keep you going strong:

1. Jelly Babies or other jelly sweets
2. Mini flapjacks
3. Dates and dried fruits
4. Mixed nuts
5. Babybels or other wrapped portions of cheese
6. Biscuits
7. Mini pork pies
8. Peanut butter and jam sandwiches
9. Salty pretzels
10. Crisps

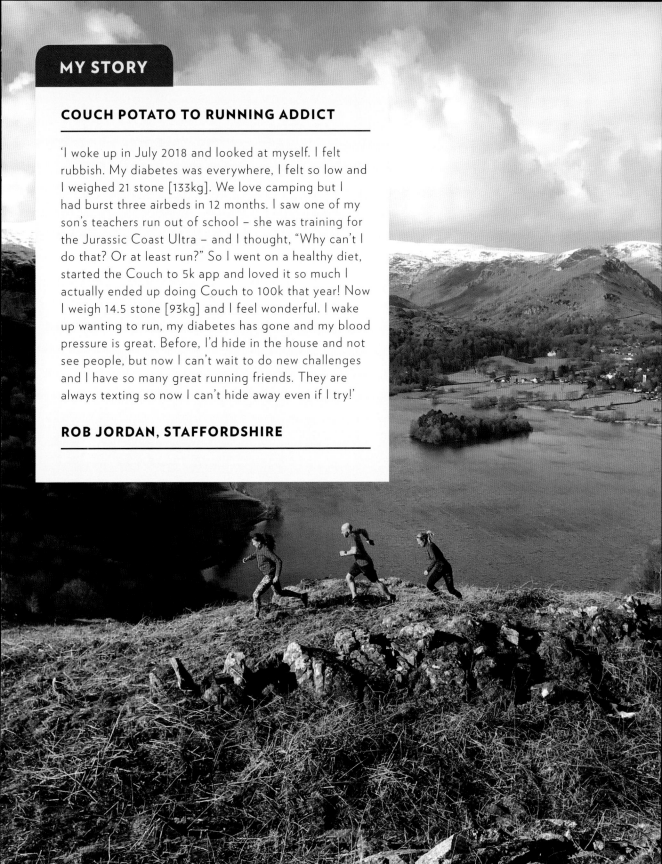

MY STORY

COUCH POTATO TO RUNNING ADDICT

'I woke up in July 2018 and looked at myself. I felt rubbish. My diabetes was everywhere, I felt so low and I weighed 21 stone [133kg]. We love camping but I had burst three airbeds in 12 months. I saw one of my son's teachers run out of school – she was training for the Jurassic Coast Ultra – and I thought, "Why can't I do that? Or at least run?" So I went on a healthy diet, started the Couch to 5k app and loved it so much I actually ended up doing Couch to 100k that year! Now I weigh 14.5 stone [93kg] and I feel wonderful. I wake up wanting to run, my diabetes has gone and my blood pressure is great. Before, I'd hide in the house and not see people, but now I can't wait to do new challenges and I have so many great running friends. They are always texting so now I can't hide away even if I try!'

ROB JORDAN, STAFFORDSHIRE

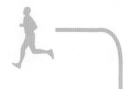

STAY MOTIVATED

One thing that has really surprised me when speaking to elite trail runners is that many of them are not super motivated all of the time – especially when the weather is bad and they feel tired from a full day of work and family commitments. The difference? They know how good they'll feel afterwards, or they have a key race in mind, so they do it anyway. Here are some tricks to help us mere mortals do the same.

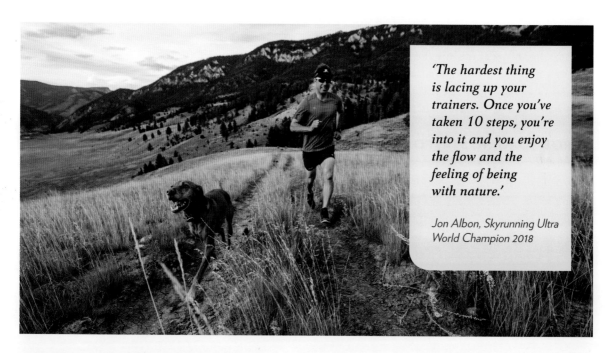

> *'The hardest thing is lacing up your trainers. Once you've taken 10 steps, you're into it and you enjoy the flow and the feeling of being with nature.'*
>
> Jon Albon, *Skyrunning Ultra World Champion 2018*

WATCH AN INSPIRATIONAL FILM
It might be raining outside, or cold, or you could be tired, so watch a short running film on YouTube to give you the motivation to get going.

RUN WITH FRIENDS
Make a commitment to run with a friend and neither of you will want to let the other down. Joining a club also has the same effect, so make it fun and social.

RUN WITH A DOG
If your dog is fit enough, change a walk or two for a run, or see if someone else's dog could do with wearing out.

DIARISE IT
Commit to your run or workout by putting it in your diary and treating it as an important business meeting with your own body.

THINK ABOUT YOUR GOAL
Aim for a certain challenge, race, distance, time or charity fundraising goal to get you out of the door.

TELL POSITIVE PEOPLE
When you've decided your goal or challenge, tell the most positive people you know – their support will keep you going.

PLAY MUSIC OR PODCASTS
Get a funky, upbeat playlist or an inspirational podcast in your headphones to energise yourself before a run.

TREAT YOURSELF
Decide what workouts you want to do this month, then promise yourself a shiny new piece of kit if you complete them all.

MAKE IT ABOUT MORE THAN JUST RUNNING
Pick a race and raise money for charity, join GoodGym for physically active community projects or go plogging – litter picking on the run!

STAY CONNECTED, GET INSPIRED, STAY MOTIVATED!

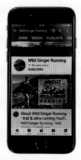

- **Read *Trail Running* magazine**
  The UK's only magazine dedicated entirely to the exciting, adventurous world of off-road running, co-founded and edited until 2017 by me!

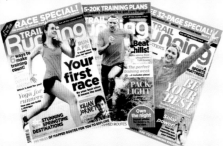

- **Watch Wild Ginger Running YouTube channel**
  Free trail and ultra running advice, inspiration, gear tests and interviews with top trail runners and expert coaches on YouTube.

- **Listen to running podcasts**
  Try Marathon Talk, Free Weekly Timed (the parkrun podcast), Talk Ultra, Tough Girl and Totally Active Podcast.

- **Follow runners on social media**
  Try following the incredible off-road athletes and coaches who give advice in quotes throughout this book. Their Instagram photos, workouts and race wins will have you reaching for your trail shoes!

- **Join running Facebook groups**
  Feel part of an online running community wherever you live. Search trail running to find your tribe, from vegan runners to gear test groups.

READ THIS EVERY TIME YOUR MOTIVATION DIPS

EXCUSE:
I don't have time

BUSTED:
Yes you do! Make time: prioritise a 30-minute run by diarising it, arranging to meet a friend or putting it at the top of your to-do list. Do this once, twice then three times a week until it becomes a habit.

EXCUSE:
I didn't sleep well

BUSTED:
Ah ha! Then running (not too late at night) will make you sleep better tonight – it's a scientific fact (*see* p. 157).

EXCUSE:
I feel depressed

BUSTED:
Many people have found running a good natural antidepressant, alleviating depression. Be kind to yourself and give it a go.

EXCUSE:
I'm not fast enough

BUSTED:
No one minds how fast you run apart from you, and anyone who makes any negative comments about your speed can quite frankly go to hell.

EXCUSE:
It's cold, dark and raining

BUSTED:
Get yourself a good head torch, a quality waterproof and some reflective gear (*see* pp. 22–23) and venture out into this exciting world of raindrops, puddles and mud.

EXCUSE:
I might get lost

BUSTED:
Maybe, but it's all part of the adventure! Turn to p. 52 to brush up on your navigation and learn the skills that will help prevent you getting lost.

GET FRIENDS AND FAMILY TRAIL RUNNING

Here are a few tips to ease your nearest and dearest into your fave sport:

• Go on a walk-run
Take those who are worried about their fitness on a walk-run, where you walk up the hills, walk and jog the flat sections, and jog the downhills.

• Watch a race
Invite people to watch a race such as parkrun, which features people of all shapes, sizes, ages and backgrounds, to inspire them.

• Tips for kids
Make it a game: see if they enjoy running in short bursts to things like trees, rocks and flowers, or cycle while you run.

• Tips for teens
If they show interest, encourage it, but for some this is not the right time for running – talk to them and see which other sports they might try for fitness and well-being.

• Tips for dogs
Make sure the breed is suited to running, wait until they are old enough and build the mileage gradually. If you intend to do canicross (running with your dog attached to you) and your dog isn't too big and strong, invest in a bungee lead secured around your waist for hands-free running.

MY STORY

HOW TO STAY MOTIVATED

'When I heard about Lowri Morgan's 333 Challenge on a podcast, I wanted to follow in her footsteps to make this my 2019 goal. Running 150 miles [240km] over the Welsh Three Peaks was going to be hard, but harder still was staying motivated for every run, including back-to-back long runs. Some days, I really struggled to get out of the door, so I would ask myself if it was because I couldn't be bothered or if I was genuinely tired and needed rest. If it was the former I'd forget what my plan said and run at least 2 miles [3.2km]. The hardest part was getting out – once in your kit it's easier to turn those 2 miles [3.2km] into 4 [6.4km], then 6 [9.6km], maybe even more. Once I'd completed double figures I could keep going. Inspirational running podcasts and audiobooks also kept me company on long runs.'

SALLY GILSON, MONMOUTH

BEING ECO-FRIENDLY

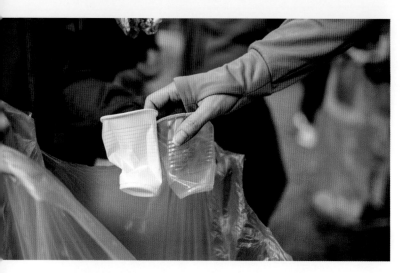

As trail runners, we love running in unspoilt, natural landscapes, so we must do all we can to protect and enhance the environment and promote sustainable, ethical working conditions worldwide.

Here are a few simple ideas you can take to the trails.

PLOGGING
This is a Swedish term for jogging while picking up litter and can be done anywhere by anyone. Make it your mission to pick up a piece of litter on every run, or take a bag with you on a dedicated clean-up mission.

BUY LESS GEAR
You need the right kit to run safely and comfortably on trails, but once you have all the items you need, ask yourself, 'Do I really need this new thing?' If the answer is 'yes', go for it! But also consider buying second-hand on Facebook groups such as Outdoor Gear Exchange or eBay and doing gear swaps with friends.

REPAIR OLD GEAR
Save money as well as the environment by getting things repaired at places such as Lancashire Sports Repairs, who will resole trail shoes and sew up holes in any kind of kit. You can also re-waterproof old jackets, sew things back together yourself or add features to your kit, like retro-fitting a strap or bungee cord to your pack so you can attach poles.

RERUN CLOTHING
Donate your and your friends' unwanted running clothes to ReRun, who will upcycle it (chop it up and make it look cool) and sell it via their community website to help reduce carbon, water and waste footprints by 20–30 per cent each. It's run by Team GB 24hr Ultra runner Dan Lawson and family. https://rerunclothing.org/

REDUCE RACE T-SHIRTS
Dan Lawson from ReRun Clothing says, 'Currently 70 per cent of donations are race T-shirts, many of which are unworn. Imagine if together we could change that.' To reduce plastic (polyester), they

ask runners to email race organisers to suggest they don't create race T-shirts or give runners the option when they enter.

WASH LESS!

If your running clothes don't smell bad after your run, wear them again! Every time you don't wash a 5kg (11lb) load, you save nearly 440kg (970lb) CO_2 emissions, plus water and detergent savings. Hang clothes to dry rather than tumble drying and save water by challenging yourself to only take five-minute showers. Look for clothing treated with Polygene or similar bacteria-beating technology so there's less smell and less need for washing.

FLYING

Trail running is an exciting way to see the world, as you will find out from the overseas race ideas in chapter 7, but you are probably already aware that it has the largest carbon footprint compared to any other mode of transport. Flying less, taking boats, trains and lift-sharing is the only sure way to tackle your conscience on this one. However, obviously that's often not possible, so consider donating to a trusted carbon-offsetting scheme. www.ethicalconsumer.org

LIFT-SHARING

Many races have a Facebook group so it's worth seeing if you can lift-share. If the race doesn't have a group, make a suggestion to the race organiser so you can start the eco-ball rolling.

USE YOUR OWN CUP

Many trail races require runners to carry their own cup rather than using single-use plastic cups,

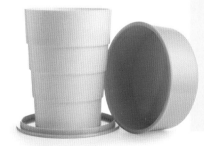

to save on landfill and reduce ocean plastic. Take your own lightweight, multi-use plastic cup or use your water bottle.

PATH MAINTENANCE

Many races donate to local path maintenance projects and charities to offset the erosion caused by footfall and some even require competitors to complete a certain amount of hours of path maintenance before they enter. Suggest this to race organisers and look for path projects with charities such as Fix the Fells, The Conservation Volunteers (TCV), GoodGym, The Land Trust, The Woodland Trust and the National Trust.

SPREAD THE WORD

Word of mouth is a powerful tool for change, so let's gently and joyfully encourage our friends and running club to adopt these eco-friendly ideas too.

MY STORY

THREE PIECES OF PLASTIC

'I started 3POP (Three Pieces of Plastic) in 2018 because I wanted to do my bit with keeping plastic out of the sea and beautiful mountainsides on the Isle of Man where I live. I pick up at least three pieces on every run and I've joined forces with Beach Buddies and A Life Less Plastic to organise community initiatives like beach cleans. We can all do our bit on every run.'

RICHARD MACNEE, ISLE OF MAN

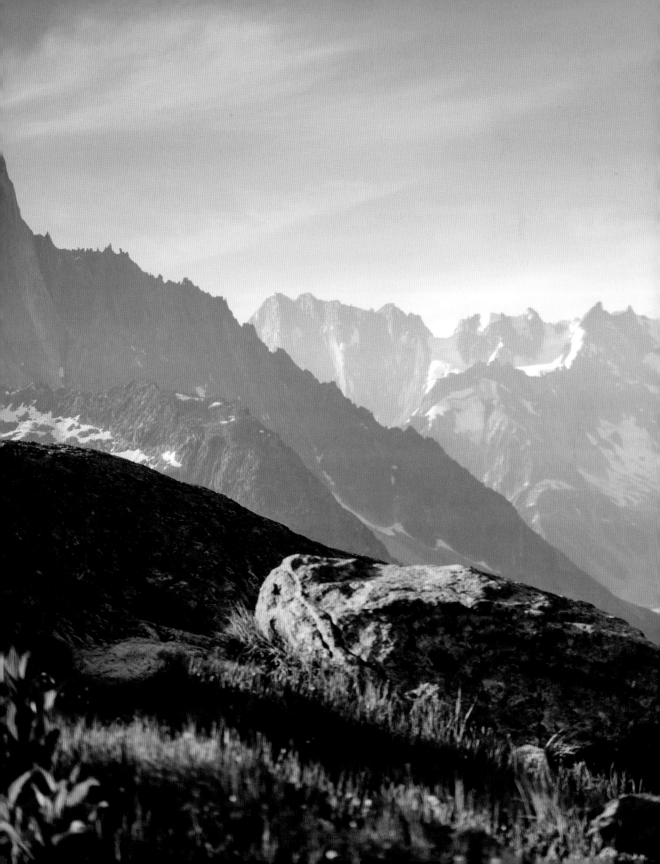

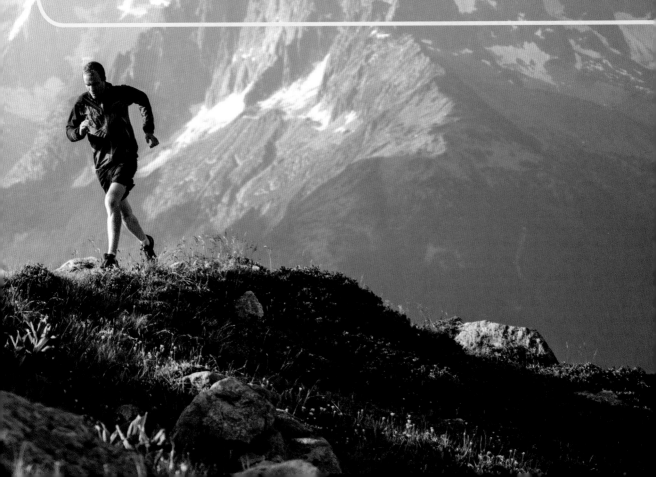

SKILLS AND TECHNIQUES

With off-road running there are some unique skills and techniques to hone, like dealing with uneven terrain, hills, weather and even peeing outdoors. This chapter will give you the confidence to tackle trails like a pro.

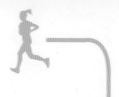

HOW TO FIT RUNNING IN

Juggling work, kids, family, a social life and other hobbies can seem like a logistical nightmare, but here are a few tricks to guarantee you fit that run into your busy day.

SWAP SOCIAL MEDIA FOR RUNNING

If you lose hours to social media, put a time limit on your phone or have social media detox days. If you can't stay away, remember it's far more important to do the run first, take piccies, upload your story, then browse everyone else's afterwards.

THE 45-MINUTE TRICK

Go to bed 45 minutes earlier than usual, then get up 45 minutes earlier and go for a quick run before you start your day. This gets your run done so you don't have to worry about fitting it in or stress about missing it later.

USE YOUR COMMUTE

A commute is a powerful way to combine running with a journey you have to make anyway. If your commute is too long to run, go by bike – it's great for mental variety and injury prevention. If your commute is very long, can you park halfway and run in? Or ride in and get a lift back? If there aren't showers at your workplace, ask them why not. Maybe there's a nearby gym with showers?

DON'T SIT DOWN!

If the only time you have to run is after work, ban yourself from sitting down when you get through the door and have your kit laid out ready to get changed into.

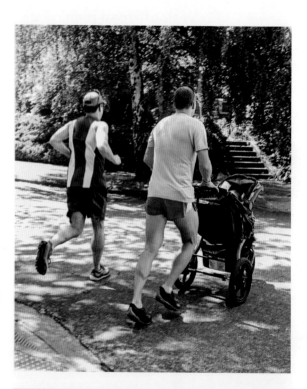

'I time my heating to come on a few hours after home time so I don't come back to a temptingly warm house and sink into the sofa. This saves me money too!'

Ben Mounsey, teacher and Team Inov8 athlete

WEAR RUNNING KIT

If you have a day full of errands or taxiing the kids to various activities, put on your running kit so the moment you get 30 minutes of freedom you don't waste time thinking, 'Shall I bother getting changed and doing my run?'

GET FIT ANYWHERE

Turn to p. 66 for a fantastic strength workout you can do absolutely anywhere, even a hotel room.

RUNNING BUGGY FITNESS

You may have seen parents pushing buggies at parkruns, races and around the park, but did you know that you can also do more strenuous sessions while your baby naps? New mum and 2019 Spine Race outright winner Jasmin Paris parked her buggy halfway up a hill so she could still do her hill interval training (see p. 45).

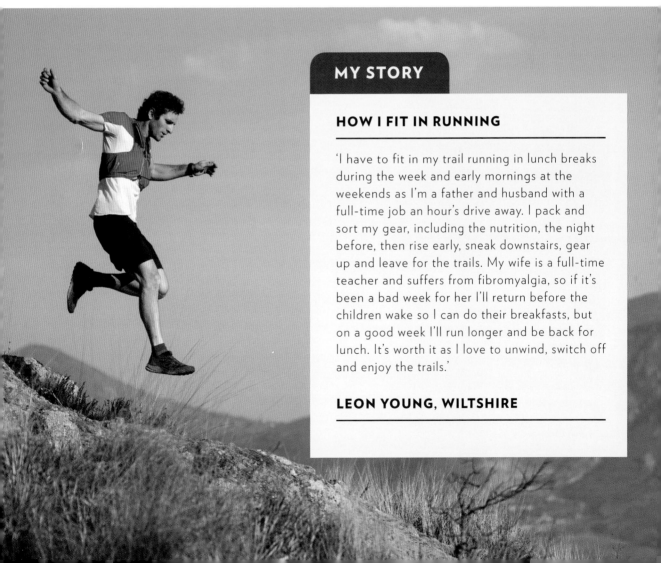

MY STORY

HOW I FIT IN RUNNING

'I have to fit in my trail running in lunch breaks during the week and early mornings at the weekends as I'm a father and husband with a full-time job an hour's drive away. I pack and sort my gear, including the nutrition, the night before, then rise early, sneak downstairs, gear up and leave for the trails. My wife is a full-time teacher and suffers from fibromyalgia, so if it's been a bad week for her I'll return before the children wake so I can do their breakfasts, but on a good week I'll run longer and be back for lunch. It's worth it as I love to unwind, switch off and enjoy the trails.'

LEON YOUNG, WILTSHIRE

HOW TO ENJOY RUNNING MORE

Of course, it will be a challenge at times, but overall, most runs should make you feel good and leave you wanting to go out more rather than collapsing in a heap saying 'Never again!' Here are some ideas to take the pressure off 'training' and harness the pure joy of trail running.

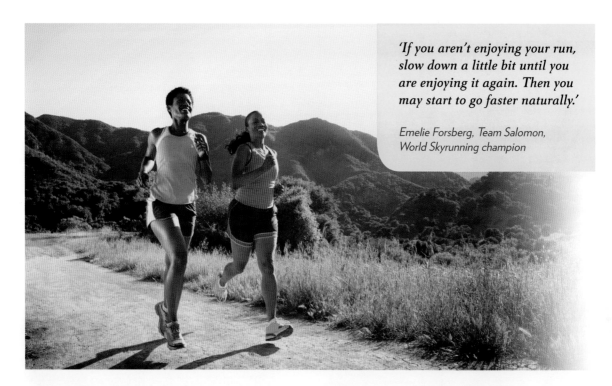

'If you aren't enjoying your run, slow down a little bit until you are enjoying it again. Then you may start to go faster naturally.'

Emelie Forsberg, Team Salomon, World Skyrunning champion

FARTLEK
Make your usual run much more exciting by doing a session invented by the Swedes. Fartlek means 'speed play' and involves running in a more childlike manner based on how you feel. You might sprint to a bench, jog to the top of a hill, hurtle down to jump over a stream, leap over a log, sprint to another tree and so on.

INTRODUCE A BEGINNER
Reignite your passion by introducing a newbie or road runner to your favourite trail routes. You'll enjoy pointing out all the cool things you pass and see the trails through their eyes, making it a win-win for both of you.

MARSHAL A RACE

Volunteer as a marshal at your local parkrun or an aspirational trail race. Seeing others achieve their goals and enjoying themselves out on the course will have you feeling like you want to run again in no time. You might even get a free entry for the next race.

JOIN GOODGYM

Doing good on your run with kind, like-minded people can't fail to invigorate you. GoodGym is a nationwide club of runners who meet up and run to physical community work projects, such as footpath maintenance for the National Trust, DIY for mental health charities and painting at old people's homes.

DO IT NAKED!

Made you look! This doesn't mean actually naked, it means without technology, be that an app on your smartphone or a fitness watch. Once you relinquish these rulers and stop stressing about pace, speed and distance, you can get back to looking at the views, concentrate on your breath and enjoy being able to run and move your body.

TRY A NEW CHALLENGE

Reverse your route, run on a new path, learn to navigate, work on a weakness – pick something new and exciting that reignites your passion for trails.

TAKE A BREAK

Sometimes, a sign of not enjoying your running is that you've overdone it. You might have overtrained (see p. 115) or be fatigued mentally and want a break from running or a change of sport. Have a rest until you're yearning to run again. If you've got energy but not for running, try something else! I've always fancied trampolining...

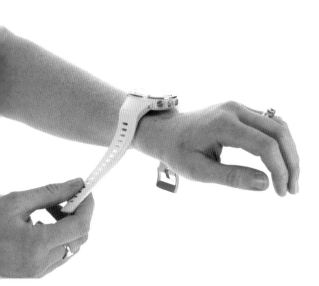

TRAIL HACK

IT'S NOT ALL ABOUT SPEED

The first thing most beginners want to know is how to get faster, but just like music, trail running isn't always better for going faster. You don't always want to listen to fast songs with no pauses or changes in tempo, and trail running is the same. Each route and each day is different. Run slow, run fast, have a break, look at the view. The most important thing is to enjoy being outside in nature, running on trails.

TACKLE TRAIL TERRAIN

This is one of the biggest ways trail differs from road running, making it much more exciting and surprising. Trails can vary from easy gravel tracks to boggy, rocky paths criss-crossed with tree roots, so here's how to deal with different terrain.

GRAVEL TRACK
Slow down gradually, and take corners and downhills with less speed and more caution as gravel can act like ball bearings underfoot.

SLIPPERY GRASS
Grippy trail shoes help to dig into slippery grass. Look for areas of more solid vegetation or rocks poking through, which can act as a stopper to prevent slippage.

TUSSOCK FIELDS
Slow down and lift your knees higher to bound over these lumps of grass, which can be as high as your waist sometimes! Relax into any slips or sinkages into the muddy field between the tussocks.

DEEP MUD
Look for patches of vegetation and rock that can provide more traction than the goop. If there are none, slow down and take smaller steps; big lunges take more energy and are likely to result in slippage.

BOG
Again, look for islands of vegetation, more solid mud, and rock to jump across. Test bog depth with a pole or tentative footstep if possible, and look for previous footsteps and animal prints that might give an indication as to whether you'll be in up to your thigh or safe not to sink.

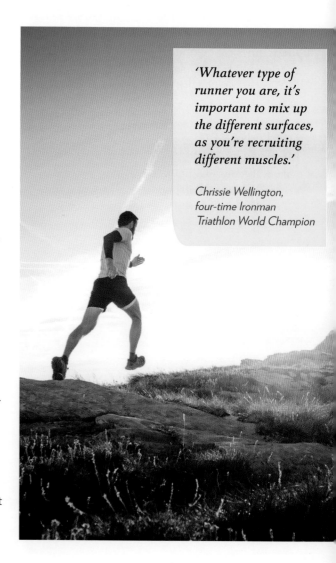

'Whatever type of runner you are, it's important to mix up the different surfaces, as you're recruiting different muscles.'

Chrissie Wellington, four-time Ironman Triathlon World Champion

TREE ROOTS

These can be treacherously slippery when wet, so tread on them with great care or step between them, if possible.

WET PLANKS

Wooden walkways over bogs and stiles often become lethally slippery when wet so slow down, take shorter steps and hold on to the fence post to cross stiles.

STEPPING STONES

Most are made of rocks that stay quite grippy even when wet, but they can become covered with slime, moss and leaves, so step with care, arms out for balance. Running poles can also help with balance.

ROCKS

These vary in slipperiness when wet or dry. Knowledge comes with experience – sometimes it's best to land on the flattest surface you can see, and sometimes it's better to plant your foot in the cracked or uneven part to avoid skidding off. With all rocky sections, think light, quick and nimble. Look ahead to pick the easiest-looking way through, slow down, take short, quick steps and don't trust either foot – expect it to slip a little and be ready for the next step.

LOOSE SCREE

This is small- to medium-sized rocks (often slate) that are not attached to the ground and slip and slide around you. Going down, treat it like skiing – relax and balance with the flow of the rocks, leaning back a little and simply sitting down if you go too fast. Going up, take short, careful steps to minimise the 'one huge step forwards, two steps back' scenario.

FRESH SNOW

This is nice to run on, reducing impact as your footprints sink into the scrunchy snow. Be prepared for some slight slipping, but go with the flow – it's usually a soft landing at least if you do fall!

HARD-PACKED SNOW

Try to run on the fresh, uncompacted snow to the sides of the path, but if there's no option, slow right down and take small steps. If this type of snow continues, it's time to put on ice grippers or spikes (see p. 161), but make sure you have the skills and experience to be in this environment safely. If not, it's best to turn round.

ICE

No one can run safely on slippery ice without ice grippers or spikes (see p. 161), so pop them on and enjoy the security of running with claws! Do make sure you are experienced enough to be in this icy environment. For example, if it's a mountainside, do you have sufficient navigation and outdoor skills? If not, it's best to turn around and go down.

TRAIL HACK

SLOW DOWN!

Look ahead; scanning the ground 2–5m (6.5–16.5ft) ahead is key to being able to react quickly. Slowing down slightly so your brain has time to process the info and send it to your feet is ironically one of the best things you can do to improve overall speed on rough ground.

MAKE UPHILLS EASIER

Trail running is often wonderfully hilly. This does mean you get fantastic views, but it is definitely more arduous. Here are some great workouts, mental tricks and technique tips to improve your speed and efficiency uphill.

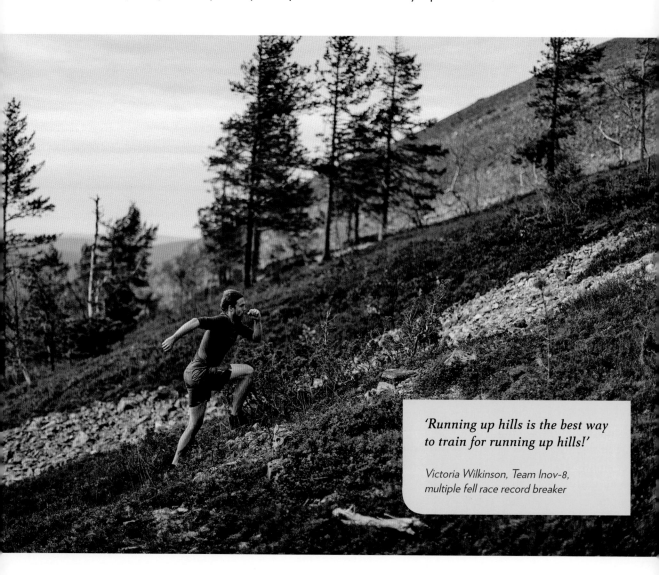

'Running up hills is the best way to train for running up hills!'

Victoria Wilkinson, Team Inov-8, multiple fell race record breaker

UPHILL TECHNIQUE

1. Lean slightly forwards from the ankles rather than at the waist.
2. Drive from the hips to feel the whole leg in action all the way up to the glutes.
3. Extend the leg fully behind you.
4. Have a short, quick stride length.
5. Drive powerfully with the arms to your sides rather than across the chest.
6. Go slower so your breathing rate doesn't get too high.
7. Find a comfortable rhythm and pace yourself.
8. Aim for trees or rocks on the way, rather than the summit.
9. Create your own small zigzags on the trail for super-steep sections.

HILL TRAINING

Also known as hill reps, uphill interval efforts will really get your heart and legs stronger and more capable. You will find plenty of this type of session in the training plans section starting p. 85. Find a runnable hill, gently sloping to start, and with a nice smooth, wide path without rocks or tussocks to trip you up. A track or even a road might be better for this in winter because it offers better traction.

HILL TRAINING ON THE FLAT

Not everyone lives near mountains, but don't worry, here are a few tricks to hill training in the most pancake flat of places.

STEP REPS

Find a set of steps or stairs and do simple or varied intervals on them instead. Add another dimension by going two steps at a time. Add squats, jumps and lunges at the top and bottom of the stairs for extra effort.

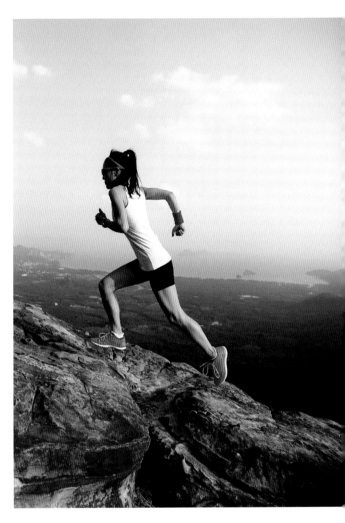

BENCH BEASTINGS

Head to a bench and create your own step aerobics class. Just make sure it's not slippery! Try:

- 20 x step-up and step-downs
- 20 x step-up and knee lifts on alternate legs
- 20 x step-up sideways with a forward leg kick
- 5 x two-legged jump-ups if the bench is the right height

MENTAL TRAINING

Getting better at hills and dreading them less is often all in the mind. Try these tricks to make hills easier:

- Remember your goal – Recall why you are doing these hill reps on this day and keep repeating it in your head. For example, say the name of a race or challenge.
- Break them down – It's tempting to look right to the top of the hill but this risks you getting disheartened. Break the hill down into sections you can run, power hike or walk to.
- Use your imagination – Imagine a top trail runner bounding powerfully up the hill in front of you, then follow them and absorb their energy.
- Choose a buzz word – Pick a powerful word such as 'strong' and think it over and over again to help you ignore tired legs and lungs and focus on your best performance.
- Shift your focus – If you get bored during hill reps, concentrate on a different aspect for improvement each time, such as technique, posture, breathing and activating your glutes.
- Talk out loud – Say 'come on' at the bottom then 'well done, four more to go' at the top to yourself or others in the group, to externalise your motivation.

TRAIL HACK

CHANGE YOUR MINDSET

I once interviewed a guy called 'Tony the Fridge' who used to run marathons with a real fridge, weighing 38kg (6 stone), strapped to his back. What's more, people put fundraising money into a slot in the top so it got heavier as the race went on! His attitude to hills under these conditions is worth remembering: 'Make friends with the hill. Be pleased to see it and welcome the challenge ahead. You are alive and you are running! Not everyone is able to do that. Thank the hill as you go up it. That positive energy will help get you to the top.'

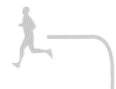

GET CONFIDENT DOWNHILL

What goes up must come down, and while downhills are thrilling for some, others can find them slightly terrifying, especially at the beginning. Here are some techniques to improve your speed and get mountain-goat confident downhill on rough ground.

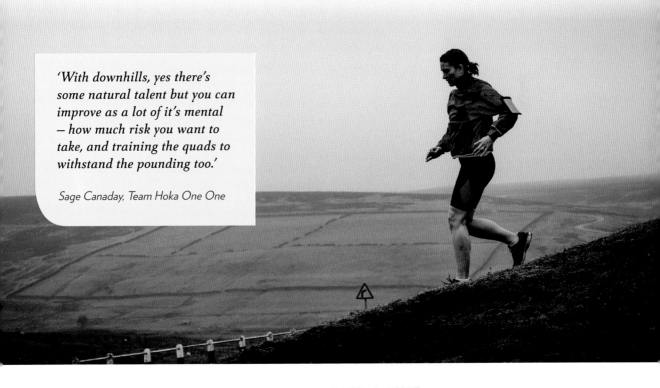

'With downhills, yes there's some natural talent but you can improve as a lot of it's mental – how much risk you want to take, and training the quads to withstand the pounding too.'

Sage Canaday, Team Hoka One One

UNEVEN TERRAIN

It's tempting to look down at your feet the whole time once the land gets lumpy, but try to keep scanning the trail from your feet to 2–5m (6.5–16.5ft) ahead. That way, your brain will have more time to process the info on the upcoming route and pass it to your feet.

PICK A LINE

When faced with a rockier or muddier section, look ahead for the easiest way across. This might involve hopping from one rock to another, or looking for flat sections or patches of vegetation that might be grippier. A good way to improve on this if you're running with others is to watch where more experienced trail runners put their feet and follow their lead.

DOWNHILL TECHNIQUE

1. Look ahead, scanning the ground for the easiest line down.
2. Neck and shoulders should be relaxed.
3. Have your arms out for balance.
4. Make sure your core is engaged and strong.
5. Constantly readjust your body position with different gradients and terrain.
6. Short, quick steps work best on tricky, broken ground.
7. Don't trust any foot excessively – always be prepared to leap to the next foot placement.
8. On easier, smoother sections, stride out without braking.

PRACTISE

The most important thing that will improve your downhill ability both physically and mentally is practise. Start with gentle, grassy slopes that won't be painful if you take a tumble. Gradually let the brakes off and relax down the hills. Head for steeper and rockier terrain as you improve at your own pace.

GET CREATIVE

If you don't live in a hilly area you can still find small ramps, slopes and steps on which to do reps. It all helps. Then try to get to a hilly or mountainous place every couple of months to put your training into practice.

LOOK AHEAD

It's tempting to look down at your feet the whole time once the land gets lumpy, but try to keep scanning the trail from your feet to 2–5m (6.5–16.5ft) ahead. This will give your brain more time to process the info on the upcoming route and pass it to your feet, so it won't be a total surprise to them.

THINK LIGHT AND RELAXED

Try to be light and springy on your feet rather than thumping down heavily, and relax into the movement, skipping and gliding down with little bounces from rock to rock, like it's a fun game. Especially relax your shoulders as they can hold a lot of tension and remember to breathe.

PICK A LINE

When faced with a more complicated-looking rocky or boggy section, look ahead for the easiest way across. This might involve hopping from one rock to another, looking for flat sections or patches of vegetation, which are often grippier than the slop they grow in.

FOLLOW SOMEONE

Someone good that is! Watch where more confident trail runners put their feet and see if you can follow their foot placements to pick up what makes a good place to land and what doesn't. If you're part of a club you could even film different runners down-hilling in slo-mo for a better look at their decisions.

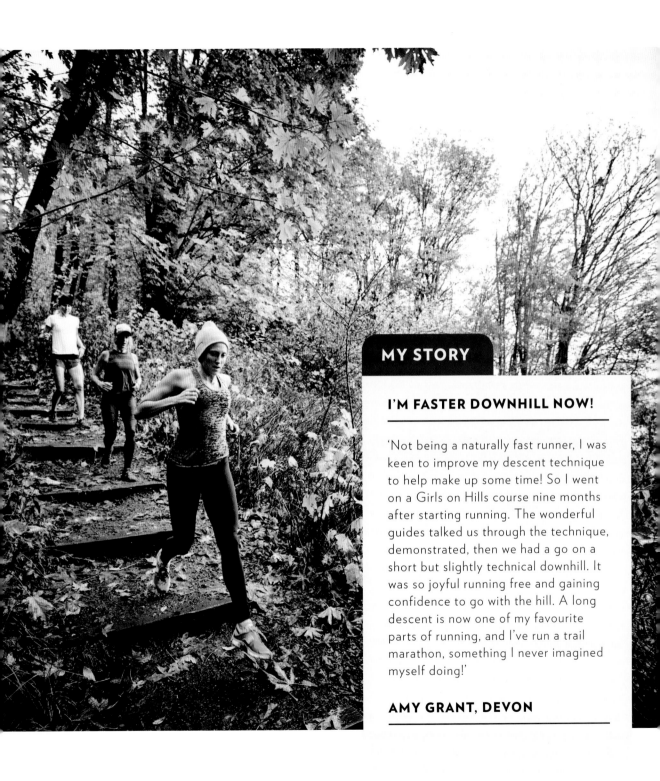

MY STORY

I'M FASTER DOWNHILL NOW!

'Not being a naturally fast runner, I was keen to improve my descent technique to help make up some time! So I went on a Girls on Hills course nine months after starting running. The wonderful guides talked us through the technique, demonstrated, then we had a go on a short but slightly technical downhill. It was so joyful running free and gaining confidence to go with the hill. A long descent is now one of my favourite parts of running, and I've run a trail marathon, something I never imagined myself doing!'

AMY GRANT, DEVON

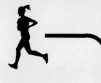

GET MORE EFFICIENT

As runners, we often always concentrate most on training our engine – the heart, legs and lungs that power you along – but actually, technique has a massive part to play in creating more efficient movement so you can run faster for longer. It's worth getting your running technique analysed by a specialist, but most of us can improve by doing the following things, according to running movement specialist and author of *The Lost Art of Running* Shane Benzie.

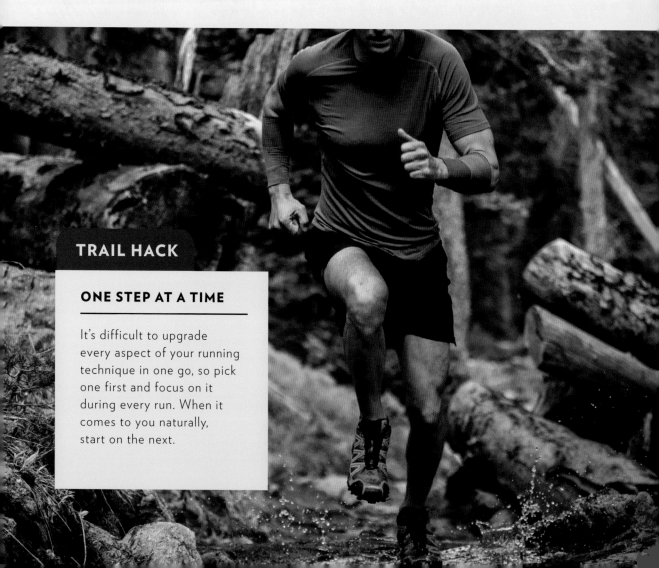

TRAIL HACK

ONE STEP AT A TIME

It's difficult to upgrade every aspect of your running technique in one go, so pick one first and focus on it during every run. When it comes to you naturally, start on the next.

1 KEEP YOUR HEAD UP

When you start getting tired on longer runs, try not to let your head drop forwards and downwards. The human head weighs 4.5kg (10lb) but for every centimetre that your head leans forwards it can feel like it weighs 1.7kg ($3^3/_4$lb) more as it puts extra stress on your spine and limits your lung capacity. So, think tall when you run – keep your head directly above your shoulders and your eyeline mainly at the horizon, looking down periodically depending on the terrain type.

2 GET THE RIGHT CADENCE

To harness the power of elastic energy from the rebound of your foot as it strikes the ground, run with a cadence (leg turnover) of 175–185 footsteps within one minute. Many new runners find this a slightly faster leg turnover than they are used to, especially if they have not done any speedwork (like intervals or tempo runs, see p. 86), but this can

also help with overstriding (landing on your heel with your foot in front of your body). Running in this cadence zone ensures that you sync in with the elastic energy you create as you make contact with the ground, which encourages a more efficient whole-foot landing rather than striking down with the heel. If your running style features long, slow strides, try shorter strides with a quicker leg turnover for a more efficient run. NB this can be more difficult on trails as your stride is always changing, but on flatter, smoother sections, this will help.

3 FOOT STRIKE

If you land on your heel and have never been injured, carry on doing your thing based on 'if it ain't broke, don't fix it' reasoning. However, Shane's research with runners has shown that rather than mid-foot striking, which became trendy in the 2010s, the most natural running stride involves a whole foot plant with heel and toe striking the ground at the same time. So if you're frequently prone to injuries or want to see if you can become more efficient and faster using a different technique, try a whole foot plant.

FIND YOUR CADENCE

Time yourself for 60 seconds while you run and count the number of times your left foot hits the ground. Double this figure to see how close you are to a 175–185 cadence zone. Some sports watches will have a cadence measure on them and also only count when one foot hits the ground, so if your watch cadence reading is around 88–92 per minute then you're on the right track. Watch the cadence film on Wild Ginger Running YouTube channel for a demo.

HOW TO WHOLE FOOT PLANT

1. Keep your whole body more upright, eyes on the horizon. Think tall, as though you're a puppet with a string fixed on top of your head and someone is pulling you up tall.
2. Take a shorter stride and focus on dropping your leg when it is directly under your hip, so your foot falls under your hip rather than striding out ahead of your body.
3. Plant the whole of your foot down at the same time rather than rolling from the heel or hitting the ground with your tiptoes.

USING A MAPPED ROUTE

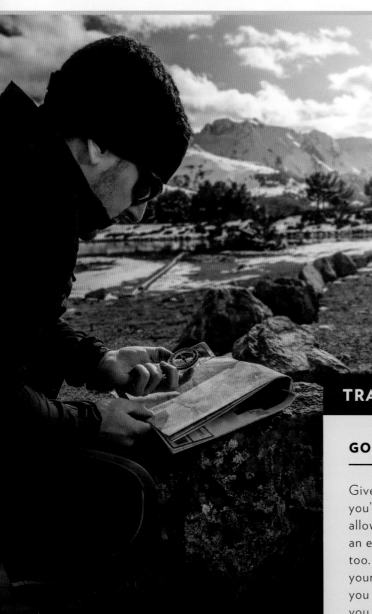

You can find fantastic trail running route maps online and in magazines such as *Trail Running*, then all it takes are a few basic map-reading skills to be able to follow them with confidence. However, I've always thought it is tricky to learn navigation from reading an explanation. I find it much easier if someone shows me how, so along with these top tips I would always recommend trying to find a good navigation course or going out on the trail with someone more experienced so you can learn from them and hone your skills.

TRAIL HACK

GO SLOW!

Give yourself more time running a route you've never navigated before, just to allow for stopping to look at the map. Take an extra layer and snack for this reason too. Always stop or slow down to confirm your location and direction. However fast you are, running the wrong way won't get you there any sooner. Stop at the top of hills and rises if possible for a view of surrounding features to help you get your bearings and work things out.

Q: Why bother with navigation skills?

A: Planning and navigating new routes using a map is much more stimulating for your brain, makes you really aware of your surroundings and takes your mind off the effort of running. Being a good navigator is essential for running safely in remote mountains and it's also a great equaliser for the super fit vs the slow plodders. You can complete a route faster by running slowly the right way rather than haring off in the wrong direction.

Q: What about the compass?

A: A compass is useful for orientating the map to confirm you've lined yourself up with the surrounding features correctly. It's essential for orientation in mist and for taking bearings so that you run in the right direction off-path. Its sides and string also measure distance on the map. However, I haven't included compass work in here as it can confuse and put off beginners and its use is difficult to demonstrate and understand from a book. To learn more, I advise asking a compass-happy friend or going on a navigation course.

Q: Can I roam where I like?

A: The Scottish Outdoor Access Code means everyone has the right to roam anywhere on most land and inland water in Scotland as long as you behave responsibly, so remember things like not leaving litter, closing gates and keeping dogs on a lead through fields with livestock. In England and Wales, you only have the right to use the specific path or bridleway across someone's land.

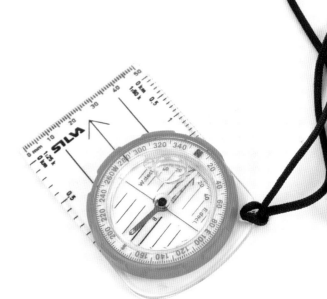

1 VITAL PREP

Before you start running, look along the route and notice any symbols, lines and patches of colour that it passes or crosses. Next, look at the legend at the edge of the map to find out what these represent in the real world. For example (most importantly!), pubs are a blue beer mug, power lines are solid black with Vs along them, and woods are green with the shape of the tree showing whether they are evergreen or deciduous. Print off or photocopy the A4 section(s) you need so you don't have to carry the whole map on your run. Pop it into a plastic folder to keep it dry so the ink doesn't run in the rain.

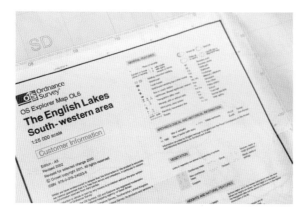

2 DIVIDE AND CONQUER

Before you start running (patience here will save you so much time while running!), divide your route into smaller sections (also known as legs) with things to look out for on the way. This is called a 'tick list' of features that you will notice and 'tick off' as you run. For example, on the first section, say to the top of a hill, you might run downhill, cross a river, turn left on the flat, then follow deciduous woodland on the right uphill for 500m (550 yards) to reach the top.

3 GET ORIENTATED

At the start of your route, orientate your map so that its features line up with what's around you in real life to help you run in the right direction. So, if you're running along a path with a river to your left, no matter whether this makes the writing on the map upside down or not, turn your map around so the river appears on the left of the path.

4 TICK OFF FEATURES

Remember the features you looked at leg by leg in point two? Now's the time to start running and ticking them off as you go. The tick list doesn't just have to be features represented by map symbols – noticing whether you should be running uphill or downhill (shown by contour lines) is one of the best tick list features as this never changes, unlike fences, land use, forestry and buildings, which can sometimes disappear, move or spring up!

5 THUMB THE MAP

As you tick your features off, keep your thumb on where you are on the map. Slide it along the route as you progress, like your sat nav locator arrow does, so you can look down at the map and quickly pinpoint where you are without having to peer at the map and work it out every time.

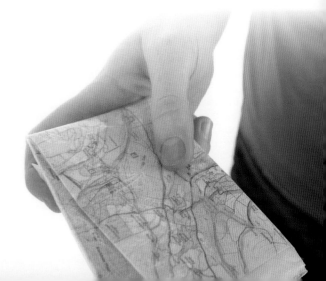

6 TIME IT

This takes a bit of practice, but as well as your features tick list, you can use timing to estimate how far you've run. If you run at a fairly even pace, you might cover say 1km (0.6 miles) in 7 minutes, so that's 500m (0.3 miles) in 3½ minutes. You can use all this info to work out when you should be looking for turns to take and features you should be passing. It also helps you not to take turns too early.

7 HAVE A CATCHING POINT

Knowing when you've run a bit too far is a very useful skill. Say you are on one path and need to take a left-hand path in 500m (0.3 miles). Having a look to see what comes just after this path will tell you when you've gone too far. Say there's a river to cross just after it, or it starts going downhill – you'll know at that point and can stop and retrace your steps before you've added another mile on.

8 ESCAPE ROUTES

Always check the forecast before you go. However, since you can never tell exactly what the weather might do or when fatigue or injury might strike, be aware of points on the route where you could safely descend, avoid a summit or rocky section, or cut the route short if needed.

EXPERT TIP

STAY SAFE!

'Check the weather before you run, especially in new, remote, exposed or high places like the hills and mountains. This will help you decide what and how much gear and food to take, but err on the side of caution and always take more rather than less. Put your waterproof/hat/ gloves on before your hands get too cold to do up the zips and push your limits gradually. Go with a more experienced friend or, better still, book a navigation or mountain skills course. Be sensible and turn back if conditions deteriorate beyond what you're comfortable with.'

JOE FAULKNER, NAVIGATION AND MOUNTAIN SKILLS INSTRUCTOR FROM NAV4 ADVENTURE

PLAN A TRAIL ROUTE

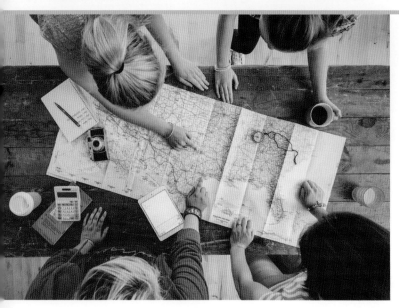

Once you've done your initial exploring using other people's trail running routes, you might be keen to plan your own with specific distances and ascent, locally or further afield. Planning a route is great fun and I enjoy poring over maps looking for interesting features and hills to run to. All you need is an Ordnance Survey (OS) or Harvey maps (waterproof walking maps) and these easy tips.

1 DECIDE ON LOCATION

Decide where you want to run and buy the OS 1:25,000 map or look at the area online in Streetmap or Bing Maps, using the 1:25,000 scale (the footpaths will show as green at this scale). OS maps also give you a code so you can access any paper map you buy from them on your computer or smartphone with their app.

2 FIND A START POINT

Look for convenient start points such as car parks, villages, visitor centres, pubs and railway stations. Ideally, these could be near to interesting features, such as cliffs, castles, monuments, lakes, forests, rivers, bridges, view points and ancient burial mounds. Familiarise yourself with the legend or key so you know what many of the symbols and features on the map mean.

3 LOOK FOR TRAILS

Look for paths and bridleways (dotted and dashed green lines) and permitted paths (dotted and dashed black lines) that connect interesting features together in order to start creating your route. One grid square is 1km (0.6 miles) in distance, so you can get a rough idea of how long your route is by laying a piece of string on your route and then measuring it against the scale, or simply roughly counting how many squares the route crosses. If you're using an app, mapping your route onto it will measure distance and ascent as you go.

4 WATCH OUT FOR HILLS!

Keep an eye on how many contour lines your route crosses and how close together they are. Contour lines are slim, brown lines curving around

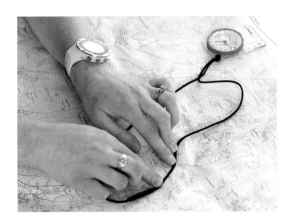

5 GET THE STATS

Using a route-making app or computer software makes this very easy, automatically telling you the distance and ascent. For old-school paper maps, use a piece of string to measure your route, then count the uphill contours the route crosses to calculate the ascent.

the map and they represent hills and valleys. You'll see numbers along them, such as 150m (492ft) and 400m (1312ft), which correspond to their height above sea level. On OS maps, they are either 5m (16.4ft) or 10m (32.8ft) apart. The closer together they are, the steeper the gradient. If your path crosses a lot of contours over a short distance it will be very steep!

TRAIL HACK

QUICK HILL TRICK

A quick trick to tell if your path runs up or downhill on a map is to look for a nearby river, as these start high and flow downhill, often getting larger as they go. Or, look for a spot height (a black dot with a number next to it indicating a measured altitude) •52 or trig point (a blue triangle with a dot in it representing a man-made stone pillar marking the top of a hill or mountain)⃤. These indicate the tops of hills or mountains.

EXPERT TIP

TOILETING OUTSIDE

'There is a general acceptance that toileting should be away from paths and watercourses, without leaving any trace, so no loo paper left – take a biodegradable dog poo bag to carry all paper and sanitary items out. Number twos should be 20–30m [66–98ft] away from watercourses – dig a hole, aim away and remember you can use leaves instead of loo paper, but spiky ones are not much fun on your delicate bum. It's never a pleasure to discover your treasure when you have a fail on the trail, so please be responsible and keep this in mind, and don't leave your poos or your paper behind.'

STUART SMITH
INTERNATIONAL MOUNTAIN LEADER FROM ADVENTURE IN MIND

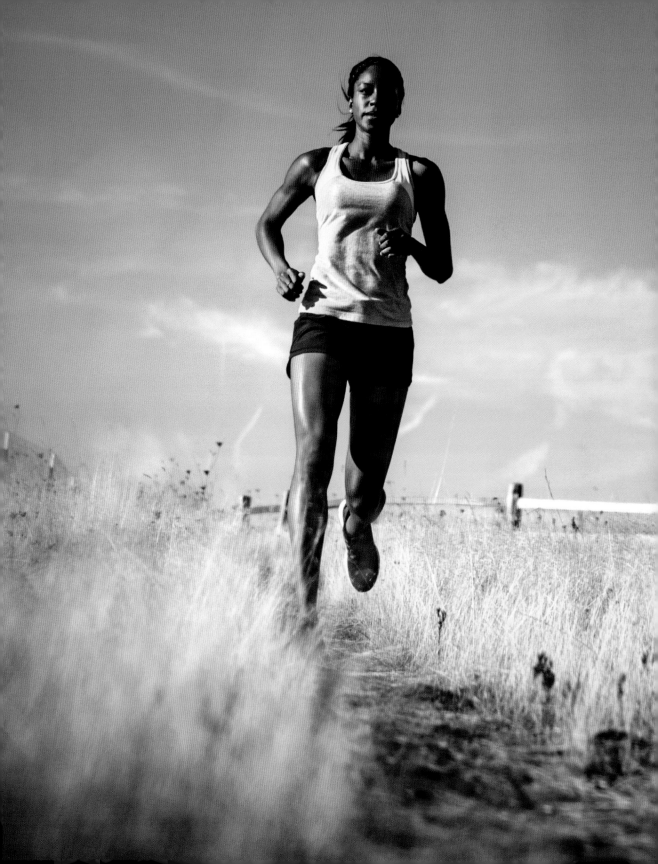

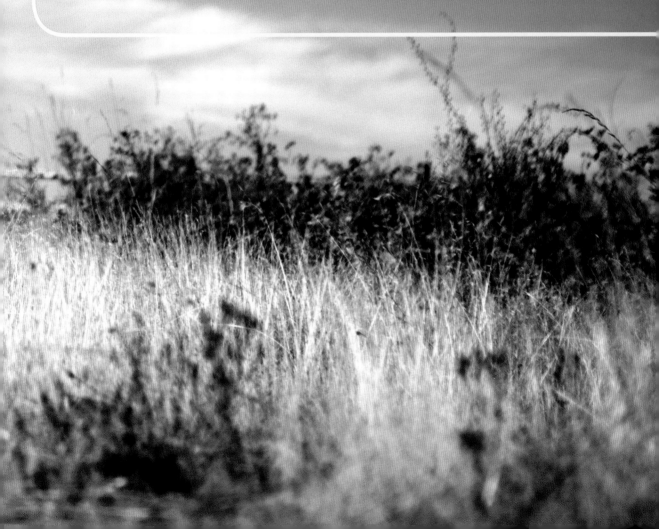

3
TRAINING AND PLANS

Many people want to improve their fitness for and performance in trail and ultra running, so whatever your current level, this chapter will explain how to get the most from your mind and body without leading to injury.

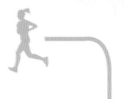

WARM UP AND COOL DOWN

To avoid injury and perform well it's always best to do a warm-up and cool-down. A warm-up is less necessary before your easy paced runs, but for fast sessions like hill reps and tempo runs (more on these later), it's essential. A cool-down routine is always helpful for quicker recovery and avoiding injury.

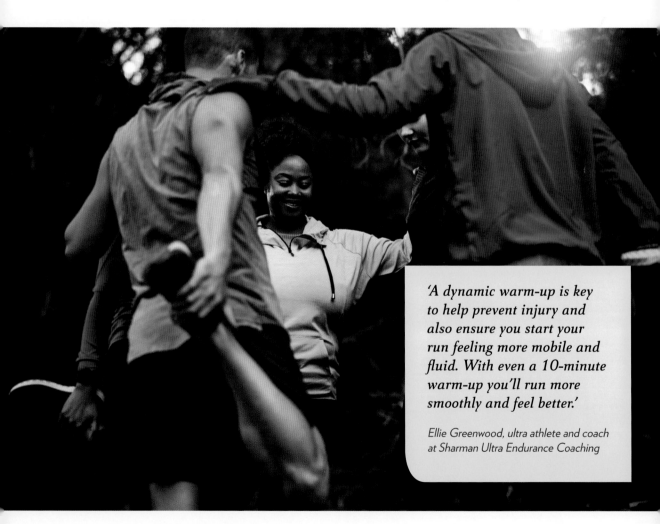

'A dynamic warm-up is key to help prevent injury and also ensure you start your run feeling more mobile and fluid. With even a 10-minute warm-up you'll run more smoothly and feel better.'

Ellie Greenwood, ultra athlete and coach at Sharman Ultra Endurance Coaching

WHY BOTHER WARMING UP?

Your muscles are a bit like Blu Tack. Imagine taking some Blu Tack straight from the fridge and trying to stretch it. What happens? It snaps. Now mould it in your hands, letting it get warm and pliable, then stretch it. Stretches like a dream! No snapping. Think of your muscles in the same way and you will never again miss your warm-up.

EASY FIVE-MINUTE WARM-UP

Start raising your pulse and mobilising the joints and muscles you will be using on your run with 10–20 seconds of the following mobility drills, interspersed with 5–10 seconds of jogging either on the spot or travelling in a circle – this is also good in a group as people can follow the leader.

Mobility Drills

1 HEEL KICKS

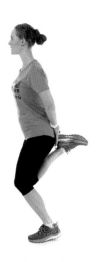

Place the back of your hands on your butt cheeks and raise your heels up to meet them.

2 KNEE RAISES

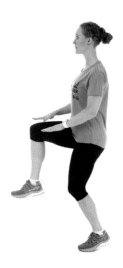

Put your hands out in front, palms down and raise your knees up high, to 90 degrees if you can, to meet them.

3 ELBOW TO OPPOSITE KNEE

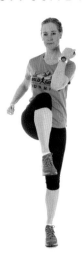

Wake up the brain with some co-ordination and mobilise the core with a twist here, lifting alternate legs to meet their opposite elbow.

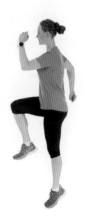

4 SKIPPING AND BOUNDING

Enjoy bouncing along with each skip and drive with the arms to aid your movement. Bounding is like skipping, but try to leap as far and high as you can to really wake up those legs and test their elastic rebound.

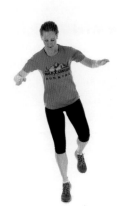

5 CLOCKWORK ANKLES

Imagine a clock face on the ground and hop clockwise from 12 o'clock to 3 o'clock to 6 o'clock to 9 o'clock on each foot. Now do it going anticlockwise. Then freestyle it! Use both feet together if you are worried about your ankles.

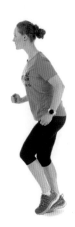

6 FAST FEET

Run on the spot quickly with fast feet, going at a moderate speed for 10 seconds, fast for 10 seconds, then count down from 10 seconds while doing an all-out sprint as fast as your feet can go.

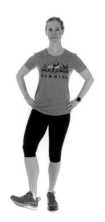

7 CIRCLES

Circle the ankles, shoulders and arms both forwards and backwards, then twist your torso left and right a few times to finish your warm up.

COOL DOWN

Allow your heart rate to slow down with 5 mins of jogging or walking. Then put on warm clothes and/or get inside if you can. Then stretch all the major muscle groups, holding each for 30-40 seconds. The stretch should be comfortable not painful – pain is telling you you are stretching too far, so ease off. Stretching regularly will lengthen your muscles and allow them a wider range of movement. Choose 5-6 stretches (see right) depending on what feels tight, covering all of them by the end of each week.

TRAIL HACK

FOAM ROLLING

Foam rolling as part of your cool-down routine is a good way to work on tight muscles and increase blood flow to help them recover quicker (*see pp. 127–129*).

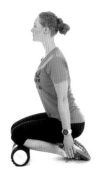

SHINS
Kneel down and place one knee on a foam roller or tightly rolled up towel with your toes pointing backwards. Gradually increase the stretch by lowering your hips to the floor.

HAMSTRINGS

QUADS (FRONT OF THE THIGHS)

CALF (GASTROCNEMIUS AND SOLEUS MUSCLES)

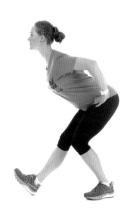

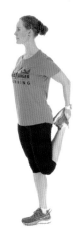

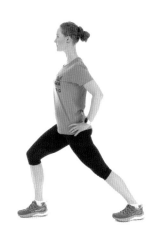

Place one leg out in front of the other, keeping the supporting leg soft at the knee (don't lock it out). Bend forwards from the hips so your chest moves forwards rather than down with a bend in your spine. Raise the toes up then down again to feel different muscles engage. Repeat on the other side.

Stand on one leg and bend the other at the knee, holding the ankle beside your bum. Keep a straight posture, shoulders up and back, knees together and thrust the hips forwards to deepen the stretch. Repeat on the other side.

Adopt a lunge position, with a straight but soft knee. This stretches the larger gastrocnemius muscle at the back of the calf. Bending the knee targets the smaller, more overlooked soleus at the side. Do both versions for 30–40 seconds each. If you can't feel the stretch, place the front of your foot on a curb or step and lower the heel slowly, again, with both a straight leg and a bent leg.

HIP FLEXORS (AROUND THE HIPS)

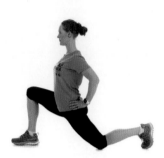

Move into a forward lunge position with the knee on the floor, keeping the chest up. Slowly bend the leading knee to feel a stretch at the front of your hips and hold for a count of 30–40 seconds. Repeat on the other side.

HIP ADDUCTORS (INNER THIGHS)

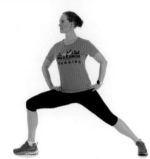

Lunge to one side, bending the leading leg, keeping the hips forwards, chest and head up. Increase the bend in the leading leg until you feel a stretch on the inside of the other leg. Hold the stretch for 30–40 seconds, then repeat on the other side.

PIRIFORMIS (DEEP IN THE BUTTOCK)

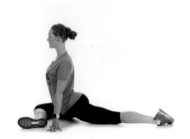

Take care if you have knee problems. Move your right leg underneath you to a near right angle, foot near your left hand. Hold for 30–40 seconds, then repeat on the other side.

GLUTES (BUTTOCKS)

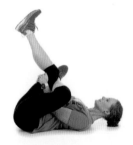

Lie down, bend both knees, then place one ankle over the other knee. Reach through the hole between your legs with one hand to clasp the other around the knee below the ankle, then pull towards your body. You can do this same move while standing up but it's harder to balance! Swap sides and repeat.

TENSOR FASCIA LATAE (TFL) (AT THE HIP)

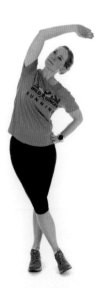

Stand up straight and cross the right leg in front of the left. Move the left foot as far to the right as it will go, stand up as straight as you can, then raise the right arm up over your head and do a side bend to the left, pushing your hips out to the right. You should feel a stretch at the front of your right hip. Hold the stretch for 30–40 seconds, then repeat on the other side.

OBLIQUES (EITHER SIDE OF YOUR TRUNK)

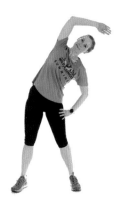

With your feet hip-distance apart, raise your right hand in the air and lean right to stretch the right side of your torso with the left hand sliding down your left thigh for balance. Hold for 30–40 seconds, then repeat on the other side.

BACK

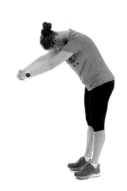

Clasp your hands and push your arms straight out in front of you, then drop your head to feel a nice stretch. Hold for 30–40 seconds. Bend over from the back to stretch out further.

CHEST

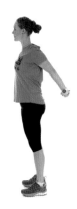

Clasp your hands behind your back, straighten your arms as much as possible and squeeze your shoulder blades together to feel a stretch across the chest. Hold for 30–40 seconds.

ARMS AND SHOULDERS

Take one arm across the chest and pull it in towards your body with the other arm, hold for 30–40 seconds, then repeat on the other side. Next, raise one arm in the air, bend at the elbow and use the other hand to gently push down on that elbow so your hand reaches further down your back. Hold for 30–40 seconds, then repeat on the other side.

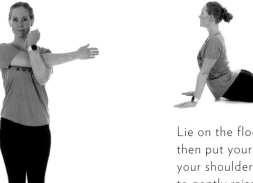

STOMACH

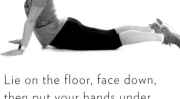

Lie on the floor, face down, then put your hands under your shoulders and use them to gently raise your head and chest upwards like a cobra.

STRENGTH FOR TRAIL RUNNERS

While it is helpful for some people, you don't *need* to get a gym membership to work on your strength if you can motivate yourself at home. Strengthen your core and whole body with this workout. Build up to doing 3 sets of 8 repetitions of each exercise with a 30-second rest between sets, starting with 1 set of 8 and adding 1 set at a time as you progress. Use a weight that's heavy enough that you are working hard to perform the move with good form on the last couple of reps of the first set, then really struggling by the third set.

TRAIL HACK

START WEIGHT-FREE

To start with, do these moves with no weights and in front of a mirror or reflective window until your form is perfect. Then add hand weights (water bottles or tins of baked beans are heavy enough at first) and/or use a running pack weighted with water bottles.

'It's important to keep your core strong because everything else works off that.'

Ricky Lightfoot, Team Salomon

STEP-UPS

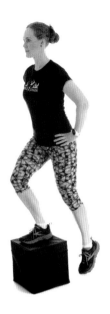

PLANK WITH MOVEMENT

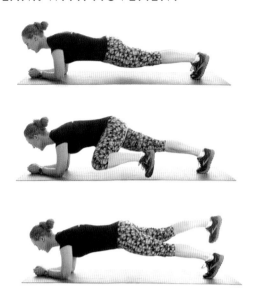

WHY?
Builds leg and glute strength and improves knee, ankle and hip stability, which is essential for trail running.

HOW?
Stand in front of a step, box or park bench and step up onto it with the whole of one foot. Bring the other foot up to stand fully on the step, then step down with the first foot and keep repeating. Do your 3 x 8 repetitions leading with this leg before swapping to lead with the other leg.

WHY?
Your core muscles are never going to be static during trail running, so adding leg and arm movements makes this move more effective.

HOW?
Get into a plank position, supporting yourself on bent elbows and tiptoes with legs straight out behind you, back straight and bum down, engaging your pelvic floor muscles (mimic stopping yourself having a wee). Now do 3 x 8 repetitions of mountain climbers on alternating legs, making sure you've done 8 repetitions on each leg in total. To do mountain climbers, bend at the knee to bring one leg as far up the side of your body as you can, then place it back into plank, then swap legs and repeat. When you've finished the mountain climbers, rest for 30 seconds. Next, move your feet hip-width apart for 3 x 8 repetitions of alternating leg lifts, again doing 8 repetitions on each side.

SQUATS AND LUNGES

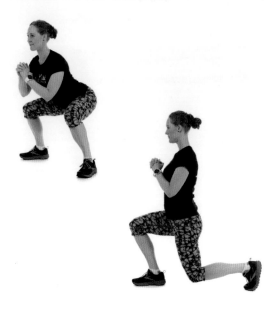

WHY?
These are fantastic strengthening moves for the entire leg and good for balance too. If you can't get to the hills, these will boost your muscle power.

HOW?
For the squat, stand with your feet shoulder-width apart, then bend the knees to drop into a squat, sticking your bum out and keeping your heels on the ground, chest and head up, looking forwards. Come back up, then do 3 x 8 repetitions. Now for the lunge. Step forwards with the right leg, bend the knees at right angles, dropping the left knee almost to the floor. Keep the chest and head up, hands on hips or arms out for balance, then rise up again. Do 3 x 8 repetitions on the same leg, then swap legs.

SINGLE-LEG SQUAT AND ARABESQUE

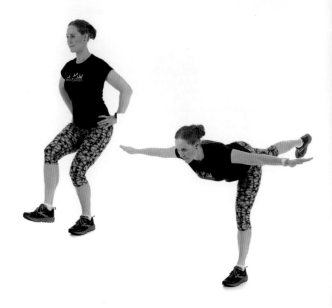

WHY?
Single-leg squats are one of the best strength exercises for runners because running is essentially a series of one-legged strength moves. The balance adds ankle stability, which is vital for uneven, rocky trails.

HOW?
Stand on one leg with your arms out to the sides for balance, keeping the knee aligned over the middle toe. Sink down slightly without knee movement from side to side (don't go deeper until you can control this), then stand up. After 3 x 8 repetitions, move into the balance. With both arms out to the side for balance, slowly lean forwards while extending the back leg straight out behind you. Hold this for five seconds while you move the arms overhead to touch the palms together and back again. Come back up to standing and repeat on the other leg.

RUSSIAN TWISTS TO V-SITS

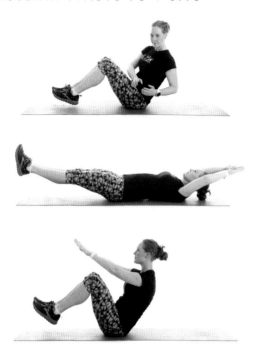

ROUND-THE-CLOCK TOE TAPS

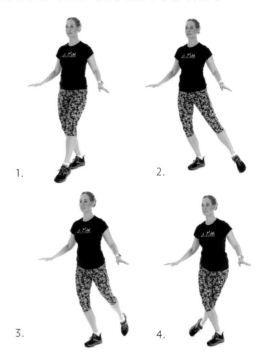

1.   2.

3.   4.

WHY?
Road running is a very straight, front-to-back activity, but trail running requires a strong torso for twisting round sudden obstacles and bends.

HOW?
Lie on a mat with your knees bent to 90 degrees, feet flat on the floor. Engage your abs, crunch up and grab a weight or your running pack. Hold it centrally above your belly and lift your feet slightly off the ground. Twist your upper body left to touch the weight almost on the ground, then the other way. That is 1 repetition. Do 3 x 8 repetitions, then move to V-sits. Straighten and lower the legs together, while at the same time raising and lowering the weight in both hands over the head. Brush the ground slightly with your hands and feet before powering back up into a sit-up position. Do 3 x 8 repetitions.

WHY?
Boosts hip flexibility, mobility, co-ordination and balance for a quicker response to fast, twisting trails.

HOW?
Stand on one leg and imagine you're at the centre of a clock face. Reach your raised foot out to the 3 o'clock position as far as you can without overbalancing. Then move it to 6 o'clock, 9 o'clock and 12 o'clock. That is 1 repetition. Do 3 x 8 repetitions before swapping to the other leg.

GLUTE BRIDGE AND LEG CIRCLES

SQUATS FOR ARMS

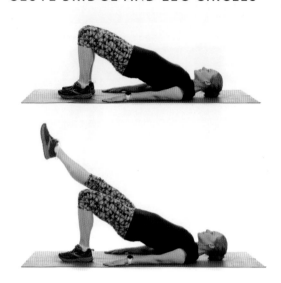

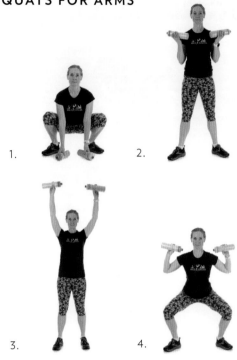

1.   2.

3.   4.

WHY?

The glutes are your body's running powerhouse so this exercise is great for strengthening them as well as increasing your core stability.

HOW?

Lie on a mat with your knees bent to 90 degrees, feet flat on the floor. Engage your pelvic floor muscles (see p. 77) and lift your hips to make a straight, diagonal line along your spine. Engage the glutes, then lift the right leg slightly and extend the leg fully. Circle it five times clockwise then five times anticlockwise, then swap the legs. This is 1 repetition. Do 3 x 8 repetitions.

WANT MORE?

For a demo of this workout and more sessions to strengthen your knees, legs, core and whole body, check out the exercise playlists on Wild Ginger Running YouTube channel.

WHY?

Trail running uses the arms a lot more than road running, since you are likely to be carrying a running pack and using poles, climbing stiles, scrambling over rocky sections and using your arms for balance.

HOW?

Stand with feet hip width apart, weights on the floor. Squat down fully, grip the weights, keep the back straight and stand up. Lift the weights up into a bicep curl, then into a shoulder press, keeping the weights either side of the ears to perform a deep squat before replacing the weights on the floor and repeating the whole sequence 3 x 8 reps.

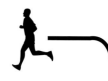

YOGA FOR TRAIL RUNNERS

Improving your balance, strength and co-ordination is great for running on uneven ground, so yoga (or Pilates) is excellent for this. Follow these moves from top trail runner and yoga enthusiast Emelie Forsberg.

CAT POSE

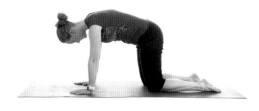

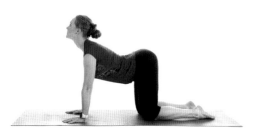

CAT POSE WITH TWIST

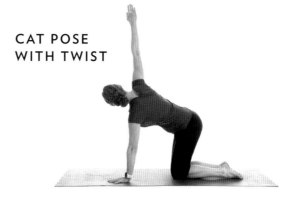

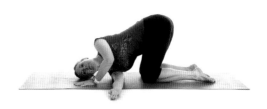

WHY?
This is a good first move to do as it loosens up and stretches the lower back and encourages deep breathing.

HOW?
On hands and knees, inhale, arch the spine and drop your head, then exhale, lower the spine and look up. Do 3–5 repetitions.

WHY?
Prepare your core for twisting trails.

HOW?
From Cat pose, raise your right arm high up in the air, twisting your upper body but keeping your hips still. Take a few breaths, then swoop this arm down through the gap between your left arm and leg, bending the left arm and coming to rest on your right shoulder. Now raise the left arm straight up into the air. Stay here for a few steady, deep breaths, then repeat on the other side.

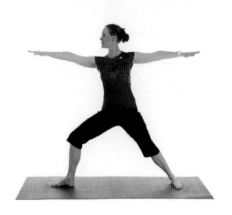

WARRIOR 2 POSE

WHY?
One to gently open the hips.

HOW?
From standing, step backwards to stand sideways with your feet wide apart and parallel. Bend the right knee and turn the left foot inwards a little. Stretch the right arm forwards and the left arm backwards, so both are parallel to the floor, looking straight ahead. Hold for a few breaths, then switch sides.

WARRIOR 3 POSE

WHY?
Time for a leg-strengthening balance.

HOW?
From Warrior 2 pose, transfer your weight forwards and straighten the leading leg. Make sure it is firmly planted and raise the back leg parallel to the floor. Stretch your arms out to either side for balance, then slowly move them into a diving position in front of your head, in line with your extended back leg. Hold for a few breaths, then lower the leg and switch sides.

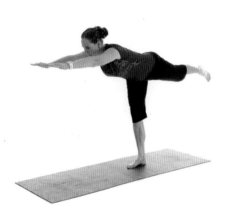

'Yoga became a complement to running, a time to stretch stiff muscles and feel how the body answered to my training.'

Emelie Forsberg, Team Salomon, World Skyrunning champion

YOGA HACK

BREATHE NATURALLY

Yoga places a lot of emphasis on the breath, but don't worry if you don't get this exactly right each time – it will start to come naturally as movements that compress the lungs prompt you to exhale and moves that open the chest out encourage you to inhale.

TRIANGLE POSE

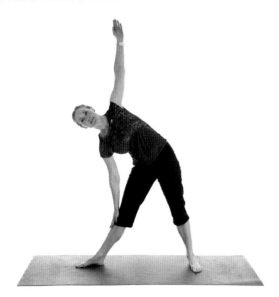

TREE POSE

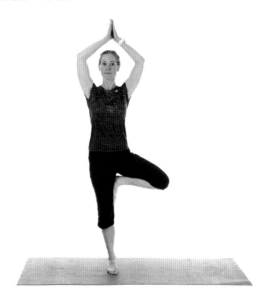

WHY?
Great for stretching each side of the body.

HOW?
From Warrior 3 pose, place the back leg back down into a stance that's slightly narrower than for Warrior 2 pose. Stand up with both arms out, one pointing forwards and the other backwards, parallel to the floor. Face the front. Exhale as you bend to the right, sliding the right hand down the leg as far as is comfortable and keeping the left arm raised straight above your head. Look up, stay for a few breaths, then change sides.

WHY?
The classic yoga balance move, great for ankle and foot strength.

HOW?
Stand up straight with your feet slightly apart and firmly planted on the ground, weight evenly distributed. Transfer your weight to your right leg and bring your left foot up so you can place the sole of the foot against your calf, inner thigh or groin (not the knee joint). Relax the shoulders and raise your arms up above your head. Hold for as many breaths as you can, then swap sides.

CROSS-TRAINING

Cross-training is extremely beneficial for all runners – mixing things up makes life even more interesting for your brain and reduces your chance of overuse and impact injuries. If you are unfortunate enough to have an injury, one of these pursuits might stop you going insane while you take a break from running.

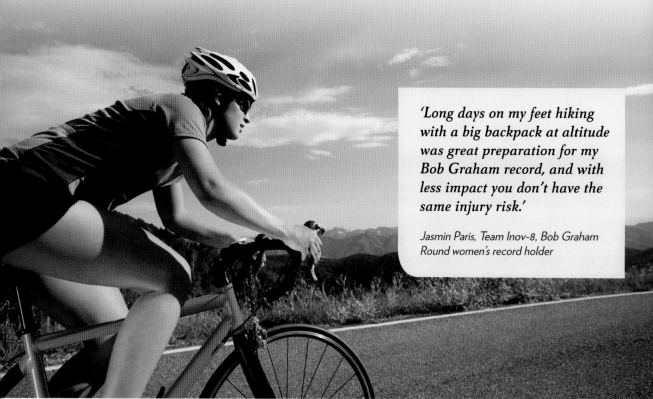

'Long days on my feet hiking with a big backpack at altitude was great preparation for my Bob Graham record, and with less impact you don't have the same injury risk.'

Jasmin Paris, Team Inov-8, Bob Graham Round women's record holder

1 STRENGTH SESSIONS

The best possible cross-training for all types of runner, giving your core and whole body the strength it needs to maintain efficient form when fatigued and to help you recover more quickly from endurance events.

2 ROAD CYCLING

A fantastic way to build leg and lung strength without the impact of running. Runners often find that despite an injury that stops them running, they can hop on the bike to maintain fitness, leg strength and sanity.

3 MOUNTAIN BIKING

Mountain biking's extra lumps and bumps compared to road cycling will give you an all-over body workout as you work hard to maintain your balance and co-ordination by using your arms and core.

4 SWIMMING

Great for the whole body, especially the breathing. Technique lessons will pay dividends for your running as you open up your lungs and learn to control your breath. A dip in a cold lake is also a fantastic way to soothe aching leg muscles after a hard run.

5 ROWING

Rowing machines are commonly found in gyms and are reasonably inexpensive to buy for your own home, and rowing with good technique on one will give your whole body an incredible workout without the impact. It's also sociable if you join a club and a boat team.

6 YOGA/PILATES

Being more flexible and having good balance is always an advantage for running on twisting, quick-changing trails. Even just 10 minutes of regular yoga or Pilates in your morning routine can improve your agility.

7 FITNESS CLASSES

Step, boxing, body pump, spinning – whatever is on offer at your local gym, have a go. Not only will these classes get you stronger and fitter, but there's also the social side – maybe convert a few people to trail running and lend them this book…?

8 HIKING

Massively underrated, hill walking is one of the best things you can do to improve your trail running endurance, uphill abilities and footwork on uneven terrain. Get more bang for your buck by hiking high-altitude mountains with a heavy backpack.

9 SCRAMBLING AND ROCK CLIMBING

Another great activity for helping you pick a line through rocky sections, scrambling (easy rock climbing, often with no ropes), rock climbing and bouldering (climbing short routes on large boulders without ropes) are great for developing core strength, flexibility and pushing your comfort zone to improve your head for heights.

10 CROSS-COUNTRY SKIING

Not available to everyone of course, but ski-racing is the long-established winter sport of many European trail runners due to the fitness benefits and whole-body workout without the impact. Your next holiday perhaps?

MY STORY

CROSS-TRAINING BOOST

'I started bouldering a few months ago, initially because it seemed fun and sociable, but I've since found the improvement in upper body strength, core strength and focus on deliberate, balanced movements has been great cross-training for trail running. It's nice to do a sport where the movement is on so many different planes, a bit different from running.'

CATHERINE DOLLIVER,
NEAR EDINBURGH

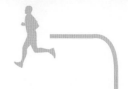

RECOVERY TIMELINE

Consider your post-workout or post-race recovery routine as the start of your next session – if you get this right, you are already improving your performance and making your next run a whole lot easier!

10 MINUTES BEFORE THE END OF EVERY TRAINING RUN

Ease into a jog and finish with a few minutes' walking to cool down and slowly bring your heart rate back down. Use this time to think about how the session went – what went well and what didn't – and what to improve for next time.

1 MINUTE AFTER

If you've worked hard at a race or had a really intense workout and there's a lake or river nearby, if it's safe enough to do so, hop in to cool your legs down and promote recovery. Then get showered or put on dry, warm clothes. You can get very cold in sweaty, wet kit even on warm days, which slows down recovery.

10 MINUTES AFTER

Stretch while your muscles are still warm. It's always better to stretch than not to, so if you end up stretching later then take things more gently as your muscles may not be quite so warm. See how on pp. 63–65.

20 MINUTES–2 HOURS AFTER

This is the ideal time to refuel after really intense runs and races more than 90 minutes long, with carbs and protein (see p. 28 for ideas). This speeds

'It's important to replace your muscles' energy stores of glycogen and the best way to do that is with chocolate milk — the perfect combination of carbs and protein. Try to stay active to keep the blood circulating, foam roll and sleep well.'

Damian Hall, UKA Coach, journalist and Team Inov-8 ultra runner

up recovery and stops you suddenly feeling famished and binging on unhealthy snacks.

30 MINUTES AFTER

After stretching, you could put on some compression tights, calf guards or socks to help promote recovery. The science behind this for performance gains isn't fully agreed, but in terms of recovery the benefits are well proven, so this is an easy way to recover faster with no effort or much movement, including on your journey home.

60 MINUTES AFTER

Lie down for five minutes with your legs at about 90 degrees in the air (against a wall or

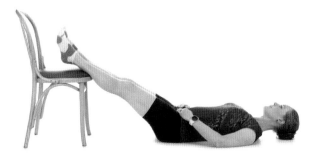

chair) every hour, if possible. This allows gravity to help your circulatory system out, returning pooled blood and flushing out lactic acid, plus it's a gentle stretch for your hamstrings.

THAT EVENING

More stretching! If you didn't get the opportunity to stretch after your run, this is better than no stretching at all and the movement will help to speed up your recovery. If it helps to pass the time, watch your favourite TV show or YouTube film and see if you can ease into some gentle stretches for 15 minutes. Be careful not to force anything as you won't be as warmed up as you were just after running. Use a foam roller too – see pp. 127–129 for the best moves.

THAT NIGHT

Sleep well. Hopefully this will come easily after running. Consistent, good-quality sleep is vital for quicker recovery and progressing your fitness. Your body will be in a state of chronic stress if not, affecting muscle repair and growth. See p. 114 for sleep advice.

MY STORY

HOW I RECOVER

'After a long, hard trail run I do a five-minute walk to keep my legs moving and to allow my heart rate to return to normal. Then it's a big drink of water and a bottle of chocolate milk. Next is a soak in a hot bath with a generous handful of Epsom salts and a large mug of tea. This really helps to soothe tired and aching muscles and wash off all that lovely mud from the trails. Then it's a refuelling meal (usually within an hour) from Anita Bean's *The Runner's Cookbook* – always tasty, with the right balance of nutrition for a faster recovery. And last but not least, a check on Strava to see how I did, because if it isn't on Strava it didn't happen!'

SIMON GEARHARDT, SURREY

THE DAY AFTER

It can be hard not to start running again immediately, but don't be tempted to squeeze in more sessions at the expense of recovery time – it's all part of training. Always follow intense or long runs and workouts with easy or rest days. Have at least one rest day per week and an easy, recovery week every month where you reduce the intensity and often the duration and frequency of training.

TRAIN RIGHT FOR YOUR AGE

As you become older, rest and recovery become even more important, but if you train right, these can be the best running years of your life – especially if you're new to the sport. As a newcomer to running, whatever your age, your performance can improve as you become more experienced, fitter and more efficient. Here's the best advice for running from your 20s to your 80s and beyond.

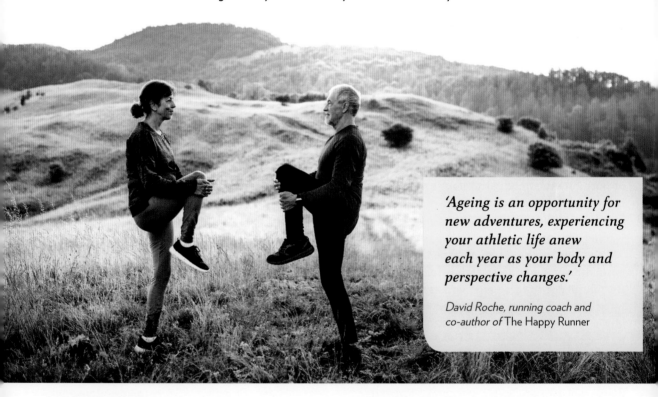

'Ageing is an opportunity for new adventures, experiencing your athletic life anew each year as your body and perspective changes.'

David Roche, running coach and co-author of The Happy Runner

IN YOUR 20S

The main risk here is burn-out as you have tons of energy and aren't afraid to use it! You might also not have developed the stamina and endurance of an older runner, so you may be best at shorter races right now. You might not even stop growing until your mid-20s, so make sure you get a lot of sleep, eat well, be aware of the signs of overtraining and get into good habits, such as stretching after you run and having a regular massage.

IN YOUR 30S

Despite there possibly being a decrease in available time due to family and work commitments in this decade, this is the prime of life for many trail runners. What you lose in strength and recovery times you gain in experience, pacing and stamina, and commitment to hard sessions like speedwork, tempo runs and hill reps. Again, though, watch out for signs of overtraining while you ride this high, and continue the stretching and regular massage.

IN YOUR 40S

So many mountain running greats are in their 40s – this decade can be the best for trail runners, especially over the longer distances, as your wisdom and experience distills into pacing, navigation skills, good fuel choices, race strategy and endurance. You may start to notice you take longer to recover and get injured more easily, so warm-ups are vital, especially before high-intensity sessions. Consider more cross-training, prioritise sleeping, good nutrition and keep up your speedwork to maintain your pace.

IN YOUR 50S

The more you stay active and ramp up your strength work, the more muscular strength you will maintain in this decade, although most runners will unfortunately start to see a decline in times. But stay positive – this could be the decade to start running further! Never neglect speedwork – you don't have to just plod along, unless you are happy with that. It's even more important to rest well, eat well, stretch, cross-train, have a regular massage and get niggles seen to before they turn into injuries.

IN YOUR 60S AND BEYOND!

Some people start running in their 70s, even their 80s, so at 60 you are still a spring chicken. If you've been running for a long time you may see old injuries rearing their ugly heads, but a good diet and rest will help with that – especially calcium-rich foods such as dairy products, nuts and dark, leafy greens. Joint supplements such as cod liver oil can also help. If you're happy running steady, go for it, but if you want to maintain your pace as much as possible, keep blasting out shorter races and training with speedwork.

EXPERT TIP

FIT FOR LIFE

'My priority now is to be fit as possible without injury. I train more consistently as work no longer gets in the way now I'm retired, so I do more cross-training and recovery. I have lost descending speed, perhaps as I am more cautious. To my 20-year-old self I'd say: plan priorities at the start of the year but be flexible – don't jeopardise your upcoming peak performance and long-term success by rushing training and racing. Cross-train to avoid overload, and rest. To conserve joints, avoid tarmac!'

WENDY DODDS, COMPLETED THE 200-MILE (320KM) DRAGON'S BACK RACE 2012, AGED 61

WOMEN'S RUNNING

There are specific hormonal changes for women that have a big impact on running and they vary enormously from woman to woman, with monthly periods, pregnancy and the menopause. There are whole books on these very important topics, but here are the essentials in a nutshell for trail runners.

'Never feel the need to apologise for who you are or how you feel. You are perfect just the way you are.'

Megan Roche, running coach and co-author of The Happy Runner

RUNNING AND MENSTRUATION

Most women can run throughout their menstrual cycle and its effect on energy levels, pain tolerance, strength and performance is finally becoming well researched. Exercise can help ease or deal with premenstrual cramps and premenstrual tension too. Using a tampon or Mooncup rather than a sanitary towel can make running more comfortable and less messy. If you have a very heavy or irregular flow, you might feel more secure using a panty liner or sanitary towel as well as a tampon.

RUNNING AND CONCEIVING

Regular exercise has been proven to increase a woman's chances of conceiving, so starting to run or continuing to do so as normal should be fine for most women trying for a baby. However, taking running to the extreme is detrimental; if you stress your body over a long period of time with hard training without enough food, you can trigger the starvation state and amenorrhea, which means your periods stop, preventing conception.

RUNNING AND PREGNANCY

Every pregnancy is different so listen to your body and run according to how you feel. Keep an open mind and be flexible. If you've never run before, pregnancy isn't the easiest time to start, but if you've made running a part of your life, run at a lower effort level until your bump becomes uncomfortable, depending on breathlessness, fatigue, pain or nausea. Keep well hydrated and ventilated, take a snack and mix running with lower-impact sports such as brisk walking, swimming and cycling. Stop running if you feel faint, dizzy, have chest pain or you have any pregnancy complications and have been advised not to run. If you have abdominal pain, bleeding or a reduction in the movement from your baby, call your emergency maternity number.

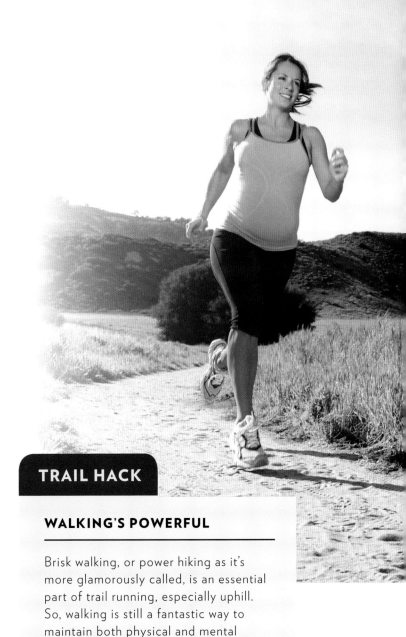

TRAIL HACK

WALKING'S POWERFUL

Brisk walking, or power hiking as it's more glamorously called, is an essential part of trail running, especially uphill. So, walking is still a fantastic way to maintain both physical and mental fitness during pregnancy.

RUNNING AND MISCARRIAGE

Sadly, miscarriage is very common, but scientific research shows it is not caused by running and exercise. One in eight pregnancies end in miscarriage according to the NHS, mostly due to abnormal chromosomes that mean the foetus is not developing as it should. After a miscarriage, the pregnancy hormones take a few weeks to go down, so you may still feel the same effects when you run. Run as soon as you like once the bleeding, cramps and any other symptoms become manageable. Be kind to yourself, ease back in only when you feel ready. Running is also great therapy for loss.

EXPERT TIP

PREGNANCY SURPRISES

'I was really surprised at how much my first trimester adversely affected my running, especially as there was no bump. I was so out of breath, like running at altitude, and I had to strap my suddenly huge boobs down with a running pack or it was too painful. Sadly, I had a miscarriage at 12 weeks, but the doctor assured me it was nothing to do with running and although I logically believe this, it is hard not to blame yourself for trying to continue as normal. During my second pregnancy (successful, yay!) I ran more steadily but also did a lot of cycling, swimming and pregnancy yoga & workouts on YouTube when the impact felt too much.'

CLAIRE MAXTED, AUTHOR

RUNNING POSTPARTUM

Again, every woman and every pregnancy is different. You hear of incredible women breastfeeding on the race finish line and expressing milk at checkpoints for 100-mile (160km) ultras, and while this is fantastic and can obviously be done, don't feel under any pressure to make this part of your journey if you're having enough of a hard time getting back to a jog. Try not to compare yourself to other running mums and return when you like; six weeks is a guideline but some mums take a year. Keep up your pelvic floor exercises and strengthen your abs as they part when the uterus expands. Avoid the plank and sit-ups while you rebuild these muscles with pelvic floor and diaphragm exercises (see p. 83).

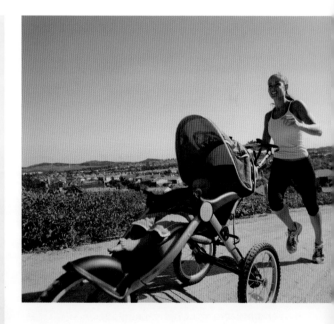

PELVIC FLOOR AND DIAPHRAGM EXERCISES

For a demo of this workout and more sessions to strengthen your knees, legs, core and whole body, check out the exercise playlists on Wild Ginger Running YouTube channel.

TOP 3 PELVIC FLOOR EXERCISES

Activate your pelvic floor at the start of each of these exercises – imagine you are stopping yourself going for a wee.

CAT COWS

Kneel on all fours, breathe in and arch your back. Hold for 3 seconds. Breathe out as you lower your back and hold again for 3 seconds. Repeat 10-15 times

SUPERMANS

Kneel on all fours, raise your right arm straight out in front and at the same time raise your left leg straight out behind you. Hold for 3-5 seconds, then back to all fours. Repeat with the other arm and leg. Do 10-15 on each side.

GLUTE BRIDGES

Lie down on your back, knees up, soles of the feet planted on the ground. Lift up your hips so you make a straight diagonal line with your torso and legs. Lift one foot off the floor to hold the whole leg out along this diagonal line. Hold for 3-5 seconds. Swap the legs. Repeat 10-15 times on each leg.

MY STORY

RUNNING AFTER A BABY

'I had an emergency C-section so I had a longer recovery period and kept active by walking our dogs. After nine weeks, I could walk 2 miles [3.2km] so I eased back into running with short distances like 5km [3.1 miles]. My tips are to agree your running routine with your partner in advance, tag team your training and accept that it doesn't always go to plan, especially during teething, bad sleep and illness. Make the most of it when you're out, doing fast sessions if you aren't out as frequently or for as long, and run with a buggy when you can. I breastfed for eight months and only realised after stopping how physically demanding it was, so trust your intuition and slow down when you need to. Now our daughter is on formula it's much easier to leave her with her dad so I can do long(ish!) runs again.'

ANNA SHAW, HAMPSHIRE

RUNNING AND THE MENOPAUSE

The menopause affects every woman differently. Hot flushes, dizziness, sleep disturbance, exhaustion, irritability, risk of osteoporosis and increased storage of fat rather than muscle formation may sound like a nightmare, but as a runner you're actually better placed to combat these symptoms. Running helps you have better sleep and moods, helps maintain bone and muscle mass and reduces fat, and you're more used to getting sweaty than non-runners! Wearing a technical, wicking vest top or T-shirt as your base layer on a run can help if you need to strip everything off to cool down during a hot flush. Listen to your body and reach out to others for tips and support.

MY STORY

RUNNING HELPS THE MENOPAUSE

'Great news, girls – running or any sport is fab for going through the menopause! It helps with the sweating and the endorphins make you feel fantastic so it helps with any tetchiness, moodiness and brain-fog. There are no downsides, and I think my symptoms weren't as bad as they could have been because of all my running. That and getting my HRT medication right after a few trips back to the doctor. So, girls, talk about the menopause, don't be embarrassed about it, and the positive side is that we don't have to worry about our period during races!'

MIMI ANDERSON,
MULTIPLE GUINNESS WORLD RECORD-BREAKING RUNNER AND ADVENTURER

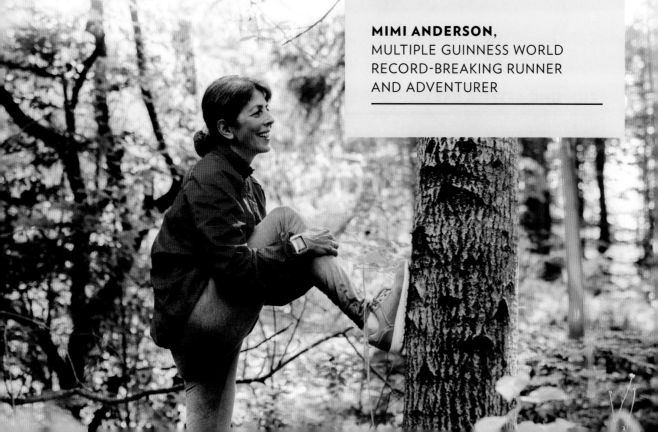

TRAINING PLANS

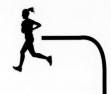

Welcome to the training zone! These plans are divided into beginner, intermediate and advanced, based on fitness rather than trail running experience, so start with the plan that is most relevant to your level. Work your way through them if increasing distance or speed is your goal, but it does not have to be – pure enjoyment is the number one aim. These plans are designed around three to five runs per week and a strength workout, but if you have time for a sixth session, mix things up with 30–60 minutes of cross-training (see pp. 74-75), such as cycling, swimming and climbing.

'There's no quick fix. Consistency is key – regular, easy running with a few harder efforts is your best performance enhancer.'

Dave Taylor, running coach from the company Fell Running Guide

IT'S COMPLICATED...

It's hard to create generic plans for trail races because courses can vary so much in terms of terrain difficulty and ascent. They range from flat – even canal towpath courses – to routes crossing several mountains over tough, scrambling ridges with a lot of hiking, not just running. Because of this, these generic plans use timing rather than distance, but you will have to be creative in how you use them depending on what your race is like. For the absolute best results, get a personalised plan from a trusted trail running coach.

A GUIDE TO EFFORT LEVELS

- **Very easy** – A very low-intensity level that means you are not out of breath at all. Used for active recovery, such as walking or very easy cycling.
- **Easy** – A comfortable pace that you can maintain for a long time and at which you can talk easily. Used for warm-ups, fun runs and long training runs.
- **Moderate** – A relatively comfortable fast pace at which you can just about still hold a conversation. Many people run every training run at this same pace, but a mix of easy and hard-paced runs is better for progression.
- **Hard** – A sustainably hard effort where you can only speak in short sentences. Used for tempo runs, longer interval efforts and some races.
- **Very hard** – A sprint speed working at maximum effort. Used for short races, sprint finishes, hill reps and any other kind of short interval efforts.

TRAINING PLAN SESSIONS EXPLAINED

FUN RUN
Have fun! Run at an easy, conversational pace, think about your form or practise hill technique, look at the views, congratulate yourself for getting out running.

STRIDES
Once a week, at the end of an easy run, practise running quicker with a few 15–20-second surges of speed with a walk back to your start point. Known as strides, these are not quite a flat-out sprint but are at a pace you can only maintain for a short time. Strides strengthen your leg muscles and get them used to a quicker turnover without overly taxing your heart and lungs.

TEMPO RUN
Great for improving your speed endurance, tempo runs should be 'comfortably hard' – at the fastest pace you can comfortably maintain for the allotted time.

HILL REPS
Reps means repetitions, and hill reps means running up the same hill again and again at speed. They're also known as hill efforts, intervals and sprints, and they're a fun way to get stronger and faster up hills, especially in a group.

STRENGTH
Stay strong and maintain good form when fatigue sets in. Use the exercises from pp. 66–70 and check out Wild Ginger Running YouTube channel exercises playlist for more workouts to strengthen your whole body.

LONG RUN
Build a strong endurance base by running longer distances at an easy pace at which you can comfortably hold a conversation. Try to replicate your race, including similar terrain and hills, which as you progress might involve travel, route planning and navigation.

YOGA
Yoga (or Pilates) is great for flexibility, balance, co-ordination, strength and also breathing and relaxation. Start with the routine on pp. 71–73.

REST
Rest is a vital part of training – this is when your body adapts to the progressively harder training load. If you overwork yourself, eventually it will catch up with you and progress will stop. Have at least one rest day per week, either totally resting or doing a very easy active recovery session such as walking.

SWAPPING SESSIONS
Move the sessions around to fit in with your week. The important thing is to make sure you have an easy or rest day after long or hard sessions such as tempo, hill reps and the long run.

TAPER
Depending on your race distance, you need to spend a certain amount of time before the event easing back from high-volume, high-intensity training so that your body is rested and raring to go on race day.

MISSED IT?
If you miss a session due to injury, illness, being busy or holidays, leave it and continue with the next week, or repeat the week if you missed a whole week. Don't try to catch up on mileage by cramming missed sessions into the following week.

BEGINNERS

BEGINNER ROAD TO TRAIL IN SIX WEEKS – 5K PLAN (SEE P. 88)

Congratulations, you already have the fitness to run 5km (3.1 miles) on roads! Maybe you have done the NHS Couch to 5k programme, or worked up to running your local parkrun. With three runs a week and a strength session, this plan will take you from 5km (3.1 miles) on roads to 5km (3.1 miles) on trails with easy skills tips as you progress.

BEGINNER 5K TO 10K TRAIL RACE IN SIX WEEKS (SEE P. 89)

Well done, you are now fit enough to run 5km (3.1 miles) on trails! This plan assumes you have just completed the transition to trail training plan, or you are fit enough from road running or other sports to start here. On three runs a week and a strength session, this plan will train you up for a beginner 10km (6.2-mile) trail race – for example, a flat or undulating route on smooth, easy trails.

TRAIL HACK

BONUS MILEAGE!

Trail races are not as strict on advertised distance as road races. If it's a mile (or five!) over, it's considered a bonus – you're getting more trails for your money.

BEGINNER TRAIL 10K TO HALF MARATHON TRAIL RACE IN NINE WEEKS (SEE P. 90)

Bravo, you can run 10km (6.2 miles) on trails! This plan assumes you have just completed the 5k to 10k trail race in six weeks training plan (see p. 89), or that you are fit enough from road running or other sports to start here. On three runs a week and a strength session, this plan will train you up for a beginner trail half marathon (13.1 miles/21.1km) – for example, a flat or undulating route on smooth, easy trails.

BEGINNER TRAIL HALF MARATHON TO TRAIL MARATHON IN 12 WEEKS (SEE P. 92)

Well done, you are able to run 13.1 miles (21.1km) – a half marathon – on trails! This plan assumes you have completed the trail 10k to half marathon trail race training plan (see p. 90) a few times, or that you are fit enough from road running or other sports to start here. This plan will train you for a beginner trail marathon (26.2 miles/42.2km) – for example, a flat or undulating route on smooth, easy trails.

BEGINNER TRAIL MARATHON TO TRAIL 50K ADD-ON (SEE P. 94)

Many trail races are only 4–5 miles (6.5–8km) over the marathon distance as they use nice round numbers such as 30 miles (48km) and 50km (31 miles). If one of these is your goal, you can use this marathon training plan, inserting this three-week block after week nine. Then continue with weeks 10, 11 and 12 to taper before your race.

	MON	TUES	WEDS	THURS	FRI	SAT	SUN	
WEEK	REST	FUN RUN	REST	FUN RUN	REST	STRENGTH	LONG RUN	MAKE IT TRAIL
1	Rest or 30 mins walk/ yoga	30 mins easy pace on easy, flat trails, 3 strides to finish	Rest or 30 mins walk/ yoga	30 mins easy pace on easy, flat trails	Rest or 30 mins walk/ yoga	Warm up 5 mins, 10 mins strength work, cool down 5 mins	30 mins easy pace on easy, flat trails	Find smooth, flat, easy paths locally, such as a canal towpath or parkland, for this transition to trails
2	Rest or 30 mins walk/ yoga	30 mins easy pace on easy, flat trails, 3 strides to finish	Rest or 30 mins walk/ yoga	35 mins easy pace on easy, flat trails	Rest or 30 mins walk/ yoga	Warm up 5 mins, 10 mins strength work, cool down 5 mins	35 mins easy pace on easy, flat trails	Pick an easy 5k trail race or work out a 5k loop locally to work towards
3	Rest or 30 mins walk/ yoga	30 mins easy pace on easy, flat trails, 6 strides to finish	Rest or 30 mins walk/ yoga	40 mins easy pace on slightly muddier, hillier trails	Rest or 30 mins walk/ yoga	Warm up 5 mins, 15 mins strength work, cool down 5 mins	40 mins easy pace on slightly muddier, hillier trails	Remember to scan the trail 2–5m (6.5–15.5ft) ahead rather than looking down at your feet
4	Rest or 30 mins walk/ yoga	30 mins easy pace on easy, flat trails, 6 strides to finish	Rest or 30 mins walk/ yoga	40 mins easy pace on slightly muddier, hillier trails	Rest or 30 mins walk/ yoga	Warm up 5 mins, 20 mins strength work, cool down 5 mins	45 mins easy pace on slightly muddier, hillier trails	Look for some slightly more challenging trails, with more mud or a few gentle hills. Walk the uphills
5	Rest or 30 mins walk/ yoga	30 mins easy pace on easy, flat trails, 6 strides to finish	Rest or 30 mins walk/ yoga	30 mins easy pace on easy, flat trails	Rest or 30 mins walk/ yoga	Warm up 5 mins, 15 mins strength work, cool down 5 mins	30 mins easy pace on easy, flat trails	Tread lightly, think about feeling springy with each step – enjoy every run!
6	Rest or 30 mins walk/ yoga	20 mins easy pace on easy, flat trails, 6 strides to finish	Rest or 30 mins walk/ yoga	20 mins easy pace on easy, flat trails	Rest or 30 mins walk/ yoga	Rest or 30 mins walk/ yoga	5k trail race or run!	Take this week very easy and you will find your race or challenge loop well within your capabilities

BEGINNER 5K TO 10K TRAIL RACE IN SIX WEEKS

	MON	**TUES**	**WEDS**	**THURS**	**FRI**	**SAT**	**SUN**	
WEEK	**REST**	**FUN RUN**	**REST**	**FUN RUN**	**REST**	**STRENGTH**	**LONG RUN**	**MAKE IT TRAIL**
1	Rest or 30 mins walk/ yoga	45 mins easy pace on slightly muddier, hillier trails, 6 strides to finish	Rest or 30 mins walk/ yoga	40 mins easy pace on slightly muddier, hillier trails	Rest or 30 mins walk/ yoga	Warm up 5 mins, 20 mins strength work, cool down 5 mins	50 mins easy pace on slightly muddier, hillier trails	Find smooth, flat, easy paths locally, such as a canal towpath or parkland, for this transition to trails
2	Rest or 30 mins walk/ yoga	45 mins easy pace on slightly muddier, hillier trails, 6 strides to finish	Rest or 30 mins walk/ yoga	45 mins easy pace on slightly muddier, hillier trails	Rest or 30 mins walk/ yoga	Warm up 5 mins, 25 mins strength work, cool down 5 mins	55 mins easy pace on slightly muddier, hillier trails	For your first trail 10km (6.2-mile), look for a race on easy paths that isn't too hilly. Go for an undulating course with smooth trails
3	Rest or 30 mins walk/ yoga	45 mins easy pace on slightly muddier, hillier trails, 6 strides to finish	Rest or 30 mins walk/ yoga	50 mins easy pace on slightly muddier, hillier trails	Rest or 30 mins walk/ yoga	Warm up 5 mins, 30 mins strength work, cool down 5 mins	60 mins easy pace on slightly muddier, hillier trails	Research at your race route and replicate the terrain and hills in your training runs as much as you can
4	Rest or 30 mins walk/ yoga	45 mins easy pace on slightly muddier, hillier trails, 6 strides to finish	Rest or 30 mins walk/ yoga	55 mins easy pace on slightly muddier, hillier trails	Rest or 30 mins walk/ yoga	Warm up 5 mins, 30 mins strength work, cool down 5 mins	65 mins easy pace on slightly muddier, hillier trails	Look for some slightly more challenging trails, with more mud or a few gentle hills. Walk the uphills, if necessary
5	Rest or 30 mins walk/ yoga	45 mins easy pace on slightly muddier, hillier trails, 6 strides to finish	Rest or 30 mins walk/ yoga	60 mins easy pace on easy, flat trails	Rest or 30 mins walk/ yoga	Warm up 5 mins, 20 mins strength work, cool down 5 mins	70 mins easy pace on easy, flat trails	Get adventurous with your long run, exploring new trails locally and further afield
6	Rest or 30 mins walk/ yoga	30 mins easy pace on easy, flat trails, 6 strides to finish	Rest or 30 mins walk/ yoga	30 mins easy pace on easy, flat trails	Rest or 30 mins walk/ yoga	Rest or 30 mins walk/ yoga	10k trail race!	Ease off this week before your first 10k trail race. These flat trails will feel so easy now!

BEGINNER TRAIL 10K TO HALF MARATHON TRAIL RACE IN NINE WEEKS

	MON	TUES	WEDS	THURS	FRI	SAT	SUN	
WEEK	REST	FUN RUN	REST	FUN RUN	REST	STRENGTH	LONG RUN	MOTIVATION
1	Rest or 30 mins walk/ yoga	60 mins easy pace on muddy trails with gentle hills, 6 strides to finish	Rest or 30 mins walk/ yoga	60 mins easy pace on muddy trails with gentle hills	Rest or 30 mins walk/ yoga	Warm up 5 mins, 30 mins strength work, cool down 5 mins	80 mins easy pace on muddy trails with gentle hills	Pick a beginner half marathon that isn't too difficult, look for undulating hills and smooth trails
2	Rest or 30 mins walk/ yoga	60 mins easy pace on muddy trails with gentle hills, 6 strides to finish	Rest or 30 mins walk/ yoga	70 mins easy pace on muddy, hilly trails	Rest or 30 mins walk/ yoga	Warm up 5 mins, 30 mins strength work, cool down 5 mins	90 mins easy pace on muddy trails with gentle hills	Look at your race route and replicate the terrain in your training runs as much as you can
3	Rest or 30 mins walk/ yoga	60 mins easy pace on muddy trails with gentle hills, 6 strides to finish	Rest or 30 mins walk/ yoga	80 mins easy pace on muddy, hilly trails	Rest or 30 mins walk/ yoga	Warm up 5 mins, 30 mins strength work, cool down 5 mins	1 hr 40 mins easy pace on muddy trails with a few steeper hills	If your race requires it, look for more challenging trails, with more mud or a few steeper hills. Walk the uphills
4	Rest or 30 mins walk/ yoga	60 mins easy pace on muddy trails with gentle hills, 6 strides to finish	Rest or 30 mins walk/ yoga	60 mins easy pace on muddy, hilly trails	Rest or 30 mins walk/ yoga	Warm up 5 mins, 30 mins strength work, cool down 5 mins	1 hr 45 mins easy pace on muddy trails with a few steeper hills	Get adventurous with your long runs, exploring new trails locally and further afield
5	Rest or 30 mins walk/ yoga	60 mins easy pace on muddy trails with gentle hills, 6 strides to finish	Rest or 30 mins walk/ yoga	70 mins easy pace on muddy, hilly trails	Rest or 30 mins walk/ yoga	Warm up 5 mins, 30 mins strength work, cool down 5 mins	1 hr 50 mins easy pace on muddy trails with a few steeper hills	Experiment with running and speed, walking up steeper hills to find out when walking is more efficient for you
6	Rest or 30 mins walk/ yoga	60 mins easy pace on muddy trails with gentle hills, 6 strides to finish	Rest or 30 mins walk/ yoga	80 mins easy pace on muddy trails with gentle hills	Rest or 30 mins walk/ yoga	Warm up 5 mins, 30 mins strength work, cool down 5 mins	1 hr 55 mins easy pace on muddy trails with a few steeper hills	Ease off this week before your first 10k trail race. These flat trails will feel so easy now!

WEEK	MON	TUES	WEDS	THURS	FRI	SAT	SUN	
	REST	**FUN RUN**	**REST**	**FUN RUN**	**REST**	**STRENGTH**	**LONG RUN**	**MOTIVATION**
7	Rest or 30 mins walk/ yoga	60 mins easy pace on muddy trails with gentle hills, 6 strides to	Rest or 30 mins walk/ yoga	60 mins easy pace on muddy trails with gentle hills	Rest or 30 mins walk/ yoga	Warm up 5 mins, 30 mins strength work, cool down 5 mins	2 hrs easy pace on muddy trails with a few steeper hills	Look for another trail race or challenge if you think you might suffer post-race blues!
8	Rest or 30 mins walk/ yoga	60 mins easy pace on muddy trails with gentle hills, 6 strides to	Rest or 30 mins walk/ yoga	70 mins easy pace on muddy trails with gentle hills	Rest or 30 mins walk/ yoga	Warm up 5 mins, 30 mins strength work, cool down 5 mins	90 mins easy pace on muddy trails with a few gentle hills	Tell friends and family you have nearly reached your goal and get their support
9	Rest or 30 mins walk/ yoga	30 mins easy pace on muddy trails with gentle hills, 6 strides to finish	Rest or 30 mins walk/ yoga	30 mins easy pace on muddy trails with gentle hills	Rest or 30 mins walk/ yoga	Rest or 30 mins walk/ yoga	Half marathon trail race!	Treat yourself to a new bit of trail running kit or another race!

A FRIENDLY WARNING!

If you are a beginner to running and/or fitness entirely, please try not to feel any pressure to run further or faster after reading this training section and all these plans. A strong endurance base takes years to build and it's more important to me that you build up gradually and gain the experience of many shorter trail races than crack out a couch to 50k. Diving in at the deep end is exciting and some may think it sounds impressive, but actually it just risks injury and burn-out. I would prefer that you spent at least a year repeating the 10k and half marathon training plans to get half a dozen of these races under your belt before spending the next year moving up to the marathon then 50k plans if distance is your aim.

BEGINNER TRAIL HALF MARATHON TO TRAIL MARATHON IN 12 WEEKS

	MON	TUES	WEDS	THURS	FRI	SAT	SUN	
WEEK	**REST**	**FUN RUN**	**REST**	**FUN RUN**	**REST**	**STRENGTH**	**LONG RUN**	**MOTIVATION**
1	Rest or 30 mins walk/ yoga	60 mins easy pace on muddy trails with gentle hills, 6 strides to finish	Rest or 30 mins walk/ yoga	60 mins easy pace on muddy trails with gentle hills	Rest or 30 mins walk/ yoga	Warm up 5 mins, 30 mins strength work, cool down 5 mins	1 hr 40 mins easy pace on muddy trails with gentle hills	Find smooth, flat, easy paths locally, such as a canal towpath or parkland, for this transition to trails
2	Rest or 30 mins walk/ yoga	60 mins easy pace on muddy trails with gentle hills, 6 strides to finish	Rest or 30 mins walk/ yoga	70 mins easy pace on muddy, hilly trails	Rest or 30 mins walk/ yoga	Warm up 5 mins, 30 mins strength work, cool down 5 mins	1 hr 50 mins easy pace on muddy trails with gentle hills	Look at your race route and replicate the trail terrain in your training runs as much as you can
3	Rest or 30 mins walk/ yoga	60 mins easy pace on muddy trails with gentle hills, 6 strides to finish	Rest or 30 mins walk/ yoga	80 mins easy pace on muddy, hilly trails	Rest or 30 mins walk/ yoga	Warm up 5 mins, 30 mins strength work, cool down 5 mins	2 hrs easy pace on muddy trails with a few steeper hills	Get adventurous with your long runs, exploring new trails locally and further afield
4	Rest or 30 mins walk/ yoga	60 mins easy pace on muddy trails with gentle hills, 6 strides to finish	Rest or 30 mins walk/ yoga	90 mins easy pace on muddy, hilly trails	Rest or 30 mins walk/ yoga	Warm up 5 mins, 30 mins strength work, cool down 5 mins	2 hrs 15 mins easy pace on muddy trails with a few steeper hills	Experiment with running and speed walking up steeper hills to find out when walking is more efficient for you
5	Rest or 30 mins walk/ yoga	60 mins easy pace on muddy trails with gentle hills, 6 strides to finish	Rest or 30 mins walk/ yoga	60 mins easy pace on muddy, hilly trails	Rest or 30 mins walk/ yoga	Warm up 5 mins, 30 mins strength work, cool down 5 mins	2 hrs easy pace on muddy trails with a few steeper hills	If you like, do a 10k trail race this weekend instead of your long run, for race experience
6	Rest or 30 mins walk/ yoga	60 mins easy pace on muddy trails with gentle hills, 6 strides to finish	Rest or 30 mins walk/ yoga	70 mins easy pace on muddy trails with gentle hills	Rest or 30 mins walk/ yoga	Warm up 5 mins, 30 mins strength work, cool down 5 mins	2 hrs 15 mins easy pace on muddy trails with a few steeper hills	Think about your race experiences to date: what prep and tactics worked best? Do more of that!

	MON	TUES	WEDS	THURS	FRI	SAT	SUN	
WEEK	REST	FUN RUN	REST	FUN RUN	REST	STRENGTH	LONG RUN	MOTIVATION
7	Rest or 30 mins walk/ yoga	60 mins easy pace on muddy trails with gentle hills, 6 strides to finish	Rest or 30 mins walk/ yoga	80 mins easy pace on muddy trails with gentle hills	Rest or 30 mins walk/ yoga	Warm up 5 mins, 30 mins strength work, cool down 5 mins	2 hrs 30 mins easy pace on muddy trails with a few steeper hills	Experiment with eating and drinking on your long runs to see what works for you
8	Rest or 30 mins walk/ yoga	60 mins easy pace on muddy trails with gentle hills, 6 strides to finish	Rest or 30 mins walk/ yoga	90 mins easy pace on muddy trails with gentle hills	Rest or 30 mins walk/ yoga	Warm up 5 mins, 30 mins strength work, cool down 5 mins	2 hrs 45 mins easy pace on muddy trails with a few gentle hills	If you like, do a half marathon trail race this weekend instead of your long run, for race experience
9	Rest or 30 mins walk/ yoga	60 mins easy pace on muddy trails with gentle hills, 6 strides to finish	Rest or 30 mins walk/ yoga	70 mins easy pace on muddy trails with gentle hills	Rest or 30 mins walk/ yoga	Warm up 5 mins, 30 mins strength work, cool down 5 mins	3 hrs easy pace on muddy trails with a few steeper hills	Check if your race has a mandatory kit list and gather the items ahead of time
10	Rest or 30 mins walk/ yoga	60 mins easy pace on muddy trails with gentle hills, 6 strides to finish	Rest or 30 mins walk/ yoga	80 mins easy pace on muddy trails with gentle hills	Rest or 30 mins walk/ yoga	Warm up 5 mins, 30 mins strength work, cool down 5 mins	2 hrs 30 easy pace on muddy trails with a few gentle hills	Look for another trail race or challenge if you think you might suffer post-race blues!
11	Rest or 30 mins walk/ yoga	60 mins easy pace on muddy trails with gentle hills, 6 strides to finish	Rest or 30 mins walk/ yoga	60 mins easy pace on muddy trails with gentle hills	Rest or 30 mins walk/ yoga	Warm up 5 mins, 30 mins strength work, cool down 5 mins	90 mins easy pace on muddy trails with a few gentle hills	Tell friends and family you have nearly reached your goal and get their support
12	Rest or 30 mins walk/ yoga	30 mins easy pace on muddy trails with gentle hills, 6 strides to finish	Rest or 30 mins walk/ yoga	30 mins easy pace on muddy trails with gentle hills	Rest or 30 mins walk/ yoga	Rest or 30 mins walk/ yoga	Marathon trail race!	Treat yourself to a new bit of trail running kit or another race or challenge!

	MON	TUES	WEDS	THURS	FRI	SAT	SUN	
WEEK	**REST**	**FUN RUN**	**REST**	**FUN RUN**	**REST**	**STRENGTH**	**LONG RUN**	**MOTIVATION**
9A	Rest or 30 mins walk/ yoga	60 mins easy pace on muddy trails with gentle hills, 6 strides to finish	Rest or 30 mins walk/ yoga	80 mins easy pace on muddy trails with gentle hills	Rest or 30 mins walk/ yoga	Warm up 5 mins, 30 mins strength work, cool down 5 mins	2 hrs 45 mins easy pace on muddy trails with a few steeper hills	Slow and steady wins the race; don't be tempted to set off too fast on these longer runs
9B	Rest or 30 mins walk/ yoga	60 mins easy pace on muddy trails with gentle hills, 6 strides to finish	Rest or 30 mins walk/ yoga	90 mins easy pace on muddy trails with gentle hills	Rest or 30 mins walk/ yoga	Warm up 5 mins, 30 mins strength work, cool down 5 mins	3 hrs easy pace on muddy trails with a few steeper hills	Check your gear fits well and doesn't chafe on these longer distances
9C	Rest or 30 mins walk/ yoga	60 mins easy pace on muddy trails with gentle hills, 6 strides to finish	Rest or 30 mins walk/ yoga	70 mins easy pace on muddy trails with gentle hills	Rest or 30 mins walk/ yoga	Warm up 5 mins, 30 mins strength work, cool down 5 mins	3 hrs 15 mins easy pace on muddy trails with a few steeper hills	Think about how far you have come since you started trail running and congratulate yourself

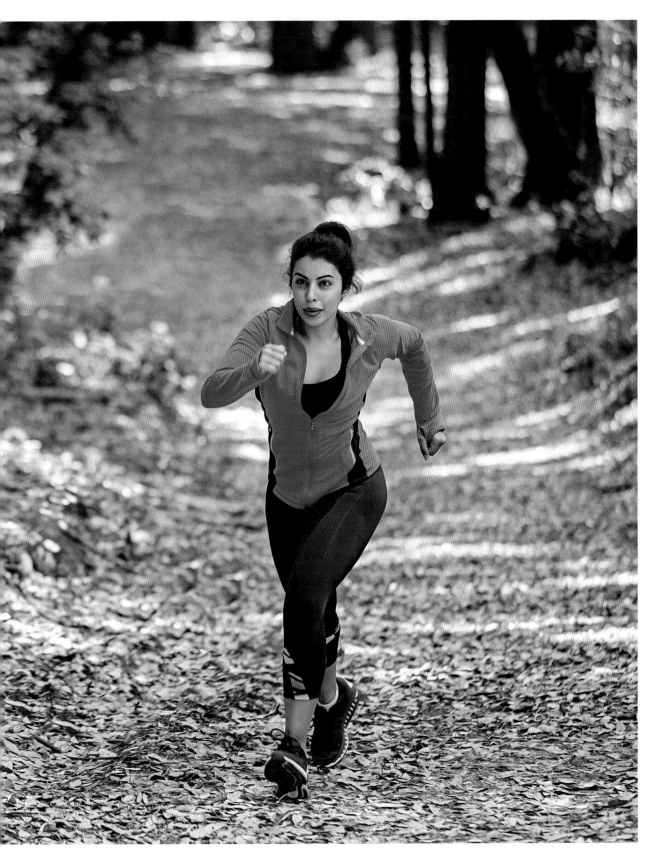

INTERMEDIATE

INTERMEDIATE 10K TRAIL RACE IN SIX WEEKS (SEE PAGE OPPOSITE)

Congratulations, you've either completed the beginner 5k–10k training plan (see p. 89) a few times now and want to get fitter, or you're fit enough from road running or other sports to dive straight into the intermediate level. This plan will prepare you for a more challenging 10k (6.2 miles) on trails with essential speed tips.

INTERMEDIATE TRAIL HALF MARATHON IN NINE WEEKS (SEE P. 98)

Time to step it up now that you've either completed the beginner trail 10k to half marathon trail race training plan (see p. 90) a few times and want to get fitter, or you're fit enough from road running or other sports to go straight into the intermediate level. This plan will prepare you for a more challenging trail half marathon (13.1 miles/21.1km) that may take three hours, with essential motivation tips.

INTERMEDIATE TRAIL MARATHON IN 12 WEEKS (SEE P. 100)

If you've made it this far then you've either completed the beginner trail half marathon to trail marathon in 12 weeks training plan (see p. 92) a few times now and want to get fitter, or you're fit enough from road running or other sports to just start at the intermediate level. This plan will prepare you for a more challenging trail marathon (26.2 miles/42.2km) that may take five to six hours.

INTERMEDIATE TRAIL MARATHON TO TRAIL 50K ADD-ON (SEE P. 102)

Many trail races are only 4 or 5 miles over the marathon distance, for example 30 miles (48km) and 50km (31 miles). Use this marathon training plan for these races by inserting this 3-week block after week 9, then complete weeks 10, 11 and 12 to taper before the race.

TRAIL HACK

MOVE SESSIONS AROUND

Always do any strength work (or rehab exercises) before a run so you are not fatigued and can perform each move with the best possible form. If you struggle to fit the easy run in on Saturday after your strength session, add it to Friday or Wednesday.

INTERMEDIATE 10K TRAIL RACE IN SIX WEEKS

	MON	TUES	WEDS	THURS	FRI	SAT	SUN	
WEEK	**REST**	**FUN RUN**	**REST**	**HILL REPS/ TEMPO RUN**	**REST**	**STRENGTH & RUN**	**LONG RUN**	**SPEED TIPS**
1	Rest or 30 mins walk/ yoga	75 mins easy pace on muddy, hilly trails, 6 strides to finish	Rest or 30 mins walk/ yoga	15 mins warm-up jog easy pace, 4 x 60-sec hill reps very hard effort, 15 mins easy jog back	Rest or 30 mins walk/ yoga	Warm up 5 mins, 40 mins strength work, cool down 5 mins. Easy run 60 mins	80 mins easy pace on trails to replicate your race	If you're new to trail running at this level, pick a race that is fully waymarked and not too rocky or hilly, to allow you time to get used to uneven terrain
2	Rest or 30 mins walk/ yoga	75 mins easy pace on muddy, hilly trails, 6 strides to finish	Rest or 30 mins walk/ yoga	15 mins warm-up jog easy pace, 15 mins tempo run hard effort, 15 mins easy jog back	Rest or 30 mins walk/ yoga	Warm up 5 mins, 40 mins strength work, cool down 5 mins. Easy run 60 mins	90 mins easy pace on trails to replicate your race	Train on trails as much as possible, only moving to road or track for the speedwork if your trails are too slippery to run fast on
3	Rest or 30 mins walk/ yoga	75 mins easy pace on muddy, hilly trails, 6 strides to finish	Rest or 30 mins walk/ yoga	15 mins warm-up jog easy pace, 6 x 60-sec hill reps very hard effort, 15 mins easy jog back	Rest or 30 mins walk/ yoga	Warm up 5 mins, 40 mins strength work, cool down 5 mins. Easy run 60 mins	1hr 40 mins easy pace on trails to replicate your race	Look at your race route and replicate the terrain in your training runs as much as you can
4	Rest or 30 mins walk/ yoga	75 mins easy pace on muddy, hilly trails, 6 strides to finish	Rest or 30 mins walk/ yoga	15 mins warm-up jog easy pace, 20 mins tempo run hard effort, 15 mins easy jog back	Rest or 30 mins walk/ yoga	Warm up 5 mins, 40 mins strength work, cool down 5 mins. Easy run 60 mins	1hr 50 mins easy pace on trails to replicate your race	Film yourself towards the end of your long run and see if your posture is still efficient, as per p. 50
5	Rest or 30 mins walk/ yoga	75 mins easy pace on muddy, hilly trails, 6 strides to finish	Rest or 30 mins walk/ yoga	15 mins warm-up jog easy pace, 8 x 60-sec hill reps very hard effort, 15 mins easy jog back	Rest or 30 mins walk/ yoga	Warm up 5 mins, 40 mins strength work, cool down 5 mins. Easy run 60 mins	60 mins easy pace on easy, flat trails	EASY WEEK Go easy this week before your 10k trail race. These flat trails will feel nice and easy.
6	Rest or 30 mins walk/ yoga	30 mins easy pace on muddy, hilly trails, 6 strides to finish	Rest or 30 mins walk/ yoga	30 mins easy pace on easy, flat trails	Rest or 30 mins walk/ yoga	Rest or 30 mins walk/ yoga	10k trail race!	Reward yourself with a trail running training camp, holiday, skills course or another race!

	MON	TUES	WEDS	THURS	FRI	SAT	SUN	
WEEK	REST	FUN RUN	REST	HILL REPS/ TEMPO RUN	REST	STRENGTH & RUN	LONG RUN	MOTIVATION
1	Rest or 30 mins walk/ yoga	75 mins easy pace on muddy, hilly trails, 6 strides to finish	Rest or 30 mins walk/ yoga	15 mins warm-up jog easy pace, 4 x 90-sec hill reps very hard effort, 15 mins easy jog back	Rest or 30 mins walk/ yoga	Warm up 5 mins, 45 mins strength work, cool down 5 mins. Easy run 60 mins	2 hrs easy pace on similar trails to your chosen race	If you're new to trail running at this level, pick a waymarked race, not too rocky or hilly, to ease yourself on to uneven terrain
2	Rest or 30 mins walk/ yoga	75 mins easy pace on muddy, hilly trails, 6 strides to finish	Rest or 30 mins walk/ yoga	15 mins warm-up jog easy pace, 20 mins tempo run hard effort, 15 mins easy jog back	Rest or 30 mins walk/ yoga	Warm up 5 mins, 45 mins strength work, cool down 5 mins. Easy run 60 mins	2 hrs 15 mins easy pace on similar trails to your chosen race	Write down why you're doing this on a Post-it note and read before every run
3	Rest or 30 mins walk/ yoga	75 mins easy pace on muddy, hilly trails, 6 strides to finish	Rest or 30 mins walk/ yoga	15 min warm up jog easy pace, 5 x 90 sec hill reps very hard effort, 15 min easy jog back	Rest or 30 mins walk/ yoga	Warm up 5 mins, 45 mins strength work, cool down 5 mins. Easy run 60 mins	2 hrs 30 mins easy pace on similar trails to your chosen race	Film yourself towards the end of your long run and see if your posture is still efficient, as per p. 50
4	Rest or 30 mins walk/ yoga	75 mins easy pace on muddy, hilly trails, 6 strides to finish	Rest or 30 mins walk/ yoga	15 mins warm-up jog easy pace, 25 mins tempo run hard effort, 15 mins easy jog back	Rest or 30 mins walk/ yoga	Warm up 5 mins, 45 mins strength work, cool down 5 mins. Easy run 60 mins	2 hrs 15 mins easy pace on similar trails to your chosen race	Watch Wild Ginger Running advice and inspiration films on YouTube for motivation
5	Rest or 30 mins walk/ yoga	75 mins easy pace on muddy, hilly trails, 6 strides to finish	Rest or 30 mins walk/ yoga	15 mins warm-up jog easy pace, 6 x 90-sec hill reps very hard effort, 15 mins easy jog back	Rest or 30 mins walk/ yoga	Warm up 5 mins, 45 mins strength work, cool down 5 mins. Easy run 60 mins	2 hrs 30 mins easy pace on similar trails to your chosen race	If possible, do a trail half marathon instead of your long run, for race experience
6	Rest or 30 mins walk/ yoga	75 mins easy pace on muddy, hilly trails, 6 strides to finish	Rest or 30 mins walk/ yoga	15 mins warm-up jog easy pace, 30 mins tempo run hard effort, 15 mins easy jog back	Rest or 30 mins walk/ yoga	Warm up 5 mins, 45 mins strength work, cool down 5 mins. Easy run 60 mins	2 hrs 45 mins easy pace on similar trails to your chosen race	PEAK WEEK Your hardest week yet. Contact your best running friends for their support

	MON	TUES	WEDS	THURS	FRI	SAT	SUN	
WEEK	REST	FUN RUN	REST	HILL REPS/ TEMPO RUN	REST	STRENGTH & RUN	LONG RUN	MOTIVATION
7	Rest or 30 mins walk/ yoga	75 mins easy pace on muddy, hilly trails, 6 strides to finish	Rest or 30 mins walk/ yoga	15 mins warm-up jog easy pace, 7 x 90-sec hill reps very hard effort, 15 mins easy jog back	Rest or 30 mins walk/ yoga	Warm up 5 mins, 45 mins strength work, cool down 5 mins. Easy run 60 mins	2 hrs easy pace on similar trails to your chosen race	Choose a piece of new trail running kit to reward yourself with in a fortnight
8	Rest or 30 mins walk/ yoga	60 mins easy pace on muddy, hilly trails, 6 strides to finish	Rest or 30 mins walk/ yoga	15 mins warm-up jog easy pace, 20 mins tempo run hard effort, 15 mins easy jog back	Rest or 30 mins walk/ yoga	Warm up 5 mins, 30 mins strength work, cool down 5 mins. Easy run 30 mins	90 mins easy pace on muddy trails with a few gentle hills	Tell friends and family you have nearly reached your goal!
9	Rest or 30 mins walk/ yoga	30 mins easy pace on muddy, hilly trails, 6 strides to finish	Rest or 30 mins walk/ yoga	30 mins easy pace on muddy trails with gentle hills	Rest or 30 mins walk/ yoga	Rest or 30 mins walk/ yoga	Half marathon trail race!	Avoid post-race blues by thinking about exciting future trail challenges

	MON	TUES	WEDS	THURS	FRI	SAT	SUN	
WEEK	REST	FUN RUN	REST	HILL REPS/ TEMPO RUN	REST	STRENGTH & RUN	LONG RUN	MOTIVATION
1	Rest or 30 mins walk/ yoga	90 mins easy pace on muddy, hilly trails, 6 strides to finish	Rest or 30 mins walk/ yoga	15 mins warm-up jog easy pace, 4 x 90-sec hill reps very hard effort, 15 mins easy jog back	Rest or 30 mins walk/ yoga	Warm up 5 mins, 45 mins strength work, cool down 5 mins. Easy run 60 mins	2 hrs 30 mins easy pace on similar trails to your chosen race	If you're new to trail running at this level, pick a waymarked race, not too rocky or hilly, to ease yourself on to uneven terrain
2	Rest or 30 mins walk/ yoga	90 mins easy pace on muddy, hilly trails, 6 strides to finish	Rest or 30 mins walk/ yoga	15 mins warm-up jog easy pace, 20 mins tempo run hard effort, 15 mins easy jog back	Rest or 30 mins walk/ yoga	Warm up 5 mins, 45 mins strength work, cool down 5 mins. Easy run 60 mins	2 hrs 45 mins easy pace on similar trails to your chosen race	Practise eating and drinking on the move during every long run
3	Rest or 30 mins walk/ yoga	90 mins easy pace on muddy, hilly trails, 6 strides to finish	Rest or 30 mins walk/ yoga	15 mins warm-up jog easy pace, 4 x 90-sec hill reps very hard effort, 15 mins easy jog back	Rest or 30 mins walk/ yoga	Warm up 5 mins, 45 mins strength work, cool down 5 mins. Easy run 60 mins	3 hrs easy pace on similar trails to your chosen race	If possible, swap your long run for a hilly half marathon trail race, for race experience
4	Rest or 30 mins walk/ yoga	60 mins easy pace on muddy, hilly trails, 6 strides to finish	Rest or 30 mins walk/ yoga	15 mins warm-up jog easy pace, 10 mins tempo run hard effort, 15 mins easy jog back	Rest or 30 mins walk/ yoga	Warm up 5 mins, 30 mins strength work, cool down 5 mins. Easy run 60 mins	5–6 hr hike in the mountains replicating the ascent of your race	EASY WEEK Watch a Wild Ginger Running trail race or run movie on YouTube
5	Rest or 30 mins walk/ yoga	90 mins easy pace on muddy, hilly trails, 6 strides to finish	Rest or 30 mins walk/ yoga	15 mins warm-up jog easy pace, 5 x 90-sec hill reps very hard effort, 15 mins easy jog back	Rest or 30 mins walk/ yoga	Warm up 5 mins, 45 mins strength work, cool down 5 mins. Easy run 60 mins	3 hrs 15 mins easy pace on similar trails to your chosen race	Make a funky, motivational playlist to listen to during or before each run
6	Rest or 30 mins walk/ yoga	90 mins easy pace on muddy, hilly trails, 6 strides to finish	Rest or 30 mins walk/ yoga	15 mins warm-up jog easy pace, 30 mins tempo run hard effort, 15 mins easy jog back	Rest or 30 mins walk/ yoga	Warm up 5 mins, 45 mins strength work, cool down 5 mins. Easy run 60 mins	3 hrs 30 mins easy pace on similar trails to your chosen race hills	Think about your race experiences to date: what prep and tactics worked best? Do more of that!

	MON	TUES	WEDS	THURS	FRI	SAT	SUN	
WEEK	REST	FUN RUN	REST	HILL REPS/ TEMPO RUN	REST	STRENGTH & RUN	LONG RUN	MOTIVATION
7	Rest or 30 mins walk/ yoga	60 mins easy pace on muddy, hilly trails, 6 strides to finish	Rest or 30 mins walk/ yoga	15 mins warm-up jog easy pace, 6 x 60-sec hill reps very hard effort, 15 mins easy jog back	Rest or 30 mins walk/ yoga	Warm up 5 mins, 30 mins strength work, cool down 5 mins. Easy run 60 mins	5–6 hr hike in the mountains replicating the ascent of your race	EASY WEEK Experiment with different gear on long runs to see what works well before the race
8	Rest or 30 mins walk/ yoga	90 mins easy pace on muddy, hilly trails, 6 strides to finish	Rest or 30 mins walk/ yoga	15 mins warm-up jog easy pace, 30 mins tempo run hard effort, 15 mins easy jog back	Rest or 30 mins walk/ yoga	Warm up 5 mins, 45 mins strength work, cool down 5 mins. Easy run 60 mins	3 hrs 45 mins easy pace on similar trails to your chosen race	If possible, swap your long run for a hilly half marathon trail race, for race experience
9	Rest or 30 mins walk/ yoga	90 mins easy pace on muddy, hilly trails, 6 strides to finish	Rest or 30 mins walk/ yoga	15 mins warm-up jog easy pace, 6 x 90-sec hill reps very hard effort, 15 mins easy jog back	Rest or 30 mins walk/ yoga	Warm up 5 mins, 45 mins strength work, cool down 5 mins. Easy run 60 mins	4 hrs easy pace on similar trails to your chosen race	PEAK WEEK Your hardest week yet. Contact your best running friends for their support
10	Rest or 30 mins walk/ yoga	90 mins easy pace on muddy, hilly trails, 6 strides to finish	Rest or 30 mins walk/ yoga	15 mins warm-up jog easy pace, 30 mins tempo run hard effort, 15 mins easy jog back	Rest or 30 mins walk/ yoga	Warm up 5 mins, 45 mins strength work, cool down 5 mins. Easy run 60 mins	3 hrs easy pace on similar trails to your chosen race	Dig out a picture of your first trail race or run to remind yourself how far you've come
11	Rest or 30 mins walk/ yoga	60 mins easy pace on muddy, hilly trails, 6 strides to finish	Rest or 30 mins walk/ yoga	15 mins warm-up jog easy pace, 6 x 60-sec hill reps very hard effort, 15 mins easy jog back	Rest or 30 mins walk/ yoga	Warm up 5 mins, 30 mins strength work, cool down 5 mins. Easy run 60 mins	2 hrs easy pace on gently hilly trails	EASY WEEK Check out all the race info, including mandatory kit, to avoid last-minute stress
12	Rest or 30 mins walk/ yoga	30 mins easy pace on muddy trails with gentle hills	Rest or 30 mins walk/ yoga	60 mins easy pace on muddy trails with gentle hills	Rest or 30 mins walk/ yoga	Rest or 30 mins walk/ yoga	Marathon trail run or race!	Did you like the marathon distance or do you prefer a 10k or half marathon? Or maybe you want to run even further...?

	MON	TUES	WEDS	THURS	FRI	SAT	SUN	
WEEK	REST	FUN RUN	REST	HILL REPS/ TEMPO RUN	REST	STRENGTH & RUN	LONG RUN	MOTIVATION
9A	Rest or 30 mins walk/ yoga	60 mins easy pace on muddy, hilly trails, 6 strides to finish	Rest or 30 mins walk/ yoga	15 mins warm-up jog easy pace, 15 mins tempo run hard effort, 15 mins easy jog back	Rest or 30 mins walk/ yoga	Warm up 5 mins, 30 mins strength work, cool down 5 mins. Easy run 60 mins	5–6 hr hike in the mountains replicating the ascent of your racehills	EASY WEEK Experiment with different nutrition now rather than during the race
9B	Rest or 30 mins walk/ yoga	90 mins easy pace on muddy, hilly trails, 6 strides to finish	Rest or 30 mins walk/ yoga	15 mins warm-up jog easy pace, 6 x 90-sec hill reps very hard effort, 15 mins easy jog back	Rest or 30 mins walk/ yoga	Warm up 5 mins, 45 mins strength work, cool down 5 mins. Easy run 60 mins	4 hrs easy pace on similar trails to your chosen race	Check your gear fits well and doesn't chafe on these longer distances
9C	Rest or 30 mins walk/ yoga	90 mins easy pace on muddy, hilly trails, 6 strides to finish	Rest or 30 mins walk/ yoga	15 mins warm-up jog easy pace, 30 mins tempo run hard effort, 15 mins easy jog back	Rest or 30 mins walk/ yoga	Warm up 5 mins, 45 mins strength work, cool down 5 mins. Easy run 60 mins	4 hrs easy pace on similar trails to your chosen race	PEAK WEEK Your hardest week yet. Slow and steady wins the race, don't be tempted to set off too fast on these longer runs

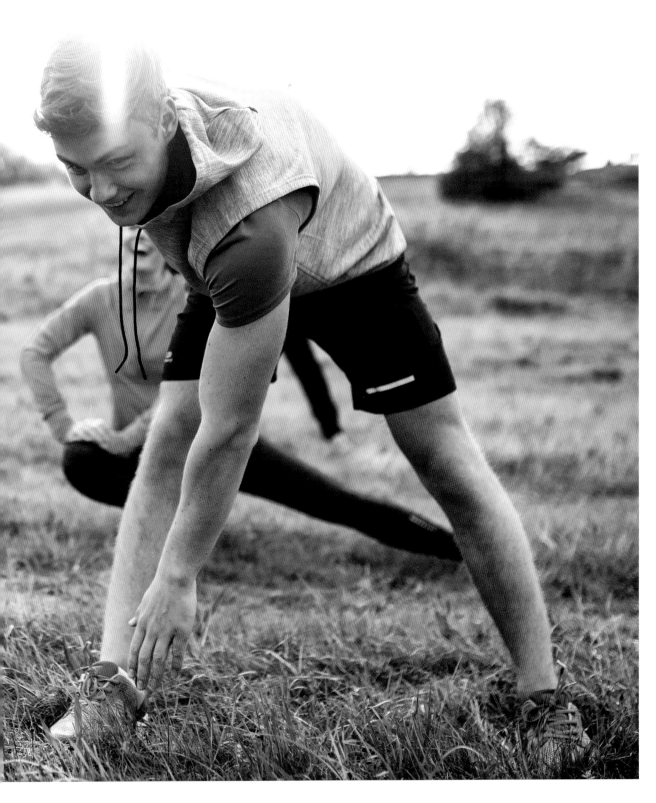

ADVANCED

ADVANCED 10K TRAIL RACE IN SIX WEEKS (SEE P. 105)

If you've reached this level then you should have either completed the intermediate 10k trail race in six weeks training plan (see p. 97) a few times and want to get fitter, or you're fit enough from road running or other sports to go straight into the advanced level. This plan will prepare you for a faster or more challenging 10km (6.2-mile) trail race.

ADVANCED TRAIL HALF MARATHON IN NINE WEEKS (SEE P. 106)

Time to amp it up. Hopefully you'll now have either completed the intermediate trail half marathon in nine weeks training plan (see p. 98) a few times or you're fit enough from road running or other sports to plunge straight into the advanced level. This plan will prepare you for a faster or more challenging half marathon trail race (13.1 miles/21.1km).

ADVANCED TRAIL MARATHON IN 12 WEEKS (SEE P. 108)

In order to do this training, you should have either completed the intermediate trail marathon in 12 weeks training plan (see p. 100) a few times or be fit enough from road running or other sports to jump straight into the advanced level. This plan will prepare you for a faster or more challenging trail marathon (26.2 miles/42.2km).

ADVANCED TRAIL 50K ADD-ON (SEE P. 110)

Use this marathon training plan for 30 miles (48km) and 50km (31-mile) races by inserting this three-week block after week nine, then complete weeks 10, 11 and 12 to taper before the race.

TRAIL HACK

MIX IT UP

If the idea of rising early to do your strength workout before parkrun in week three fills you with horror, move your strength session to Friday. Don't do it with fatigued muscles after parkrun or you risk bad form and injury.

	MON	TUES	WEDS	THURS	FRI	SAT	SUN	
WEEK	REST	FUN RUN	REST	HILL REPS/ TEMPO RUN	REST	STRENGTH & RUN	LONG RUN	SPEED TIPS
1	Rest or 30 mins walk/ yoga	75 mins easy pace on muddy, hilly trails, 6 strides to finish	Rest or 30 mins walk/ yoga	15 mins warm-up jog easy pace, 10 x 60-sec hill reps very hard effort, 15 mins easy jog back	Rest or 30 mins walk/ yoga	Warm up 5 mins, 60 mins strength work, cool down 5 mins. Easy run 60 mins	80 mins easy pace on trails to replicate your race	If you're new to trail running at this level, look for a waymarked race that isn't too rocky or mountainous to ease yourself into off-road terrain
2	Rest or 30 mins walk/ yoga	75 mins easy pace on muddy, hilly trails, 6 strides to finish	Rest or 30 mins walk/ yoga	15 mins warm-up jog easy pace, 20 mins tempo run or 5k race hard effort, 15 mins easy jog back	Rest or 30 mins walk/ yoga	Warm up 5 mins, 60 mins strength work, cool down 5 mins. Easy run 60 mins	90 mins easy pace on trails to replicate your race	Run off-road as much as possible but if it's too slippery for the fast sessions, move to road or track
3	Rest or 30 mins walk/ yoga	75 mins easy pace on muddy, hilly trails, 6 strides to finish	Rest or 30 mins walk/ yoga	15 mins warm-up jog easy pace, 6 x 60-sec hill reps & 4 x 90-sec hill reps very hard effort, 15 mins easy jog back	Rest or 30 mins walk/ yoga	Warm up 5 mins, 60 mins strength work, cool down 5 mins. Easy run 60 mins	1hr 40 mins easy pace on trails to replicate your race	Hone your hill technique during the hill rep session, focusing on good technique, as per p. 45
4	Rest or 30 mins walk/ yoga	75 mins easy pace on muddy, hilly trails, 6 strides to finish	Rest or 30 mins walk/ yoga	15 mins warm-up jog easy pace, 20 mins tempo run or 5k race hard effort, 15 mins easy jog back	Rest or 30 mins walk/ yoga	Warm up 5 mins, 60 mins strength work, cool down 5 mins. Easy run 60 mins	2 hrs 15 mins easy pace on trails to replicate race terrain & hills	Look at the hills on your race course. Where are they? What is your strategy for how hard you will push on each one?
5	Rest or 30 mins walk/ yoga	50 mins easy pace on muddy, hilly trails, 6 strides to finish	Rest or 30 mins walk/ yoga	15 mins warm-up jog easy pace, 4 x 60-sec hill reps & 6 x 90-sec hill reps very hard effort, 15 mins easy jog back	Rest or 30 mins walk/ yoga	Warm up 5 mins, 30 mins strength work, cool down 5 mins. Easy run 30 mins	60 mins easy pace on easy, flat trails	Make sure you are refuelling correctly with good-quality nutrition, especially the week before the race
6	Rest or 30 mins walk/ yoga	30 mins easy pace on muddy, hilly trails, 6 strides to finish	Rest or 30 mins walk/ yoga	60 mins easy pace on easy, flat trails	Rest or 30 mins walk/ yoga	Rest or 30 mins walk/ yoga	10k trail race!	Enjoy choosing your race reward – will it be new kit, a skills course, training camp or another race?

ADVANCED TRAIL HALF MARATHON IN NINE WEEKS

	MON	TUES	WEDS	THURS	FRI	SAT	SUN	
WEEK	**REST**	**FUN RUN**	**FUN RUN**	**HILL REPS/ TEMPO RUN**	**REST**	**STRENGTH & RUN**	**LONG RUN**	**SPEED TIPS**
1	Rest or 30 mins walk/ yoga	90 mins easy pace on muddy, hilly trails, 6 strides to finish	60 mins easy pace on easy trails	15 mins warm-up jog easy pace, 8 x 90-sec hill reps very hard effort, 15 mins easy jog back	Rest or 30 mins walk/ yoga	Warm up 5 mins, 60 mins strength work, cool down 5 mins. Easy run 60 mins	2 hrs easy pace on similar trails to your chosen race	If you're new to trail running at this level, look for a waymarked race that isn't too rocky or mountainous to ease yourself into off-road terrain
2	Rest or 30 mins walk/ yoga	90 mins easy pace on muddy, hilly trails, 6 strides to finish	60 mins easy pace on easy trails	15 mins warm-up jog easy pace, 30 mins tempo run hard effort, 15 mins easy jog back	Rest or 30 mins walk/ yoga	Warm up 5 mins, 60 mins strength work, cool down 5 mins. Easy run 60 mins	2 hrs 15 mins easy pace on similar trails to your chosen race	Run off-road as much as possible but if it's too slippery for the fast sessions, move to road or track
3	Rest or 30 mins walk/ yoga	90 mins easy pace on muddy, hilly trails, 6 strides to finish	60 mins easy pace on easy trails	15 mins warm-up jog easy pace, 6 x 2-min hill reps very hard effort, 15 mins easy jog back	Rest or 30 mins walk/ yoga	Warm up 5 mins, 60 mins strength work, cool down 5 mins. Warm up 10 mins, tempo run 20 mins or 5k race, such as parkrun	2 hrs 30 mins easy pace on similar trails to your chosen race	Video yourself in slow-mo on your smartphone to see whether your technique matches up with the top tips in this book (see p. 50)
4	Rest or 30 mins walk/ yoga	60 mins easy pace on muddy trails with gentle hills	60 mins easy pace on easy trails	15 mins warm-up jog easy pace, 10 mins tempo run hard effort, 15 mins easy jog back	Rest or 30 mins walk/ yoga	Warm up 5 mins, 30 mins strength work, cool down 5 mins. Easy run 30 mins	2 hrs easy pace on similar trails to your chosen race	EASY WEEK Refine your race strategy based on previous race performances and recce the course if you can
5	Rest or 30 mins walk/ yoga	90 mins easy pace on muddy, hilly trails, 6 strides to finish	60 mins easy pace on easy trails	15 mins warm-up jog easy pace, 4 x 3-min hill reps very hard effort, 15 mins easy jog back	Rest or 30 mins walk/ yoga	Warm up 5 mins, 60 mins strength work, cool down 5 mins. Easy run 60 mins	2 hrs 30 mins easy pace on similar trails to your chosen race	Halfway! Watch inspirational trail running films on Wild Ginger Running YouTube channel
6	Rest or 30 mins walk/ yoga	90 mins easy pace on muddy, hilly trails, 6 strides to finish	60 mins easy pace on easy trails	15 mins warm-up jog easy pace, 30 mins tempo run hard effort, 15 mins easy jog back	Rest or 30 mins walk/ yoga	Warm up 5 mins, 60 mins strength work, cool down 5 mins. Easy run 60 mins	10k trail race then 60 mins easy pace OR 2 hrs 45 mins easy pace long run	PEAK WEEK Concentrate on good form, posture, technique and breathing and continue this through to the race

WEEK	MON REST	TUES FUN RUN	WEDS FUN RUN	THURS HILL REPS/ TEMPO RUN	FRI REST	SAT STRENGTH & RUN	SUN LONG RUN	MOTIVATION
7	Rest or 30 mins walk/ yoga	90 mins easy pace on muddy, hilly trails, 6 strides to finish	60 mins easy pace on easy trails	15 mins warm-up jog easy pace, 4 x 3- min hill reps very hard effort, 15 mins easy jog back	Rest or 30 mins walk/ yoga	Warm up 5 mins, 60 mins strength work, cool down 5 mins. Easy run 60 mins	2 hrs 30 mins easy pace on similar trails to your chosen race	Decide what gear you'll race in, and make sure you have all the mandatory kit to avoid last-minute stress
8	Rest or 30 mins walk/ yoga	60 mins easy pace on muddy trails with gentle hills	60 mins easy pace on easy trails	15 mins warm-up jog easy pace, 10 mins tempo run hard effort, 15 mins easy jog back	Rest or 30 mins walk/ yoga	Warm up 5 mins, 30 mins strength work, cool down 5 mins. Easy run 30 mins	2 hrs easy pace on muddy trails with a few gentle hills	EASY WEEK Eat healthily, stay hydrated, get enough sleep and visualise yourself acing the race
9	Rest or 30 mins walk/ yoga	60 mins easy pace on muddy trails with gentle hills	Rest or 30 mins walk/ yoga	60 mins easy pace on muddy trails with gentle hills	Rest or 30 mins walk/ yoga	Rest or 30 mins walk/ yoga	Half marathon trail race!	Take it super easy in preparation for the race of your life!

	MON	TUES	WEDS	THURS	FRI	SAT	SUN	
WEEK	**REST**	**FUN RUN**	**FUN RUN**	**HILL REPS/ TEMPO RUN**	**REST**	**STRENGTH & RUN**	**LONG RUN**	**SPEED TIPS**
1	Rest or 30 mins walk/ yoga	90 mins easy pace on muddy, hilly trails, 6 strides to finish	60 mins easy pace on easy trails	15 mins warm-up jog easy pace, 8 x 90-sec hill reps very hard effort, 15 mins easy jog back	Rest or 30 mins walk/ yoga	Warm up 5 mins, 60 mins strength work, cool down 5 mins. Easy run 60 mins	2 hrs easy pace on similar trails to your chosen race	If you're new to trail running at this level, pick a waymarked race, not too rocky or hilly to ease yourself on to uneven terrain
2	Rest or 30 mins walk/ yoga	90 mins easy pace on muddy, hilly trails, 6 strides to finish	60 mins easy pace on easy trails	15 mins warm-up jog easy pace, 30 mins tempo run hard effort, 15 mins easy jog back	Rest or 30 mins walk/ yoga	Warm up 5 mins, 60 mins strength work, cool down 5 mins. Easy run 60 mins	2 hrs 30 mins easy pace on similar trails to your chosen race	Run on trails unless they're too slippery for speedwork, in which case roads and tracks are allowed!
3	Rest or 30 mins walk/ yoga	90 mins easy pace on muddy, hilly trails, 6 strides to finish	60 mins easy pace on easy trails	15 mins warm-up jog easy pace, 6 x 2-min hill reps very hard effort, 15 mins easy jog back	Rest or 30 mins walk/ yoga	Warm up 5 mins, 60 mins strength work, cool down 5 mins. Warm up 10 mins, tempo run 20 mins or 5k race, such as parkrun	3 hrs easy pace on similar trails to your chosen race	Keep a training diary to chart your progress and note what gear, nutrition, sleep and training patterns suit you best
4	Rest or 30 mins walk/ yoga	90 mins easy pace on muddy, hilly trails, 6 strides to finish	60 mins easy pace on easy trails	15 mins warm-up jog easy pace, 15 mins tempo run hard effort, 15 mins easy jog back	Rest or 30 mins walk/ yoga	Warm up 5 mins, 30 mins strength work, cool down 5 mins. Easy run 30 mins	2 hrs easy pace on similar trails to your chosen race	EASY WEEK As the long runs get longer, practise speed hiking on long/steep hills, potentially with poles
5	Rest or 30 mins walk/ yoga	90 mins easy pace on muddy, hilly trails, 6 strides to finish	60 mins easy pace on easy trails	15 mins warm-up jog easy pace, 5 x 3-min hill reps very hard effort, 15 mins easy jog back	Rest or 30 mins walk/ yoga	Warm up 5 mins, 60 mins strength work, cool down 5 mins. Easy run 60 mins	Half marathon trail race	Pick a trail half marathon similar in terrain to your marathon and really push hard. Reflect on your race strategy afterwards
6	Rest or 30 mins walk/ yoga	90 mins easy pace on muddy, hilly trails, 6 strides to finish	60 mins easy pace on easy trails	15 mins warm-up jog easy pace, 30 mins tempo run hard effort, 15 mins easy jog back	Rest or 30 mins walk/ yoga	Warm up 5 mins, 60 mins strength work, cool down 5 mins. Easy run 60 mins	3 hrs 15 mins easy pace on similar trails to your chosen race	Halfway! Keep training motivation high by watching advice-packed films on Wild Ginger Running YouTube channel

	MON	TUES	WEDS	THURS	FRI	SAT	SUN	
WEEK	REST	FUN RUN	FUN RUN	HILL REPS / TEMPO RUNS	REST	STRENGTH & RUN	LONG RUN	SPEED TIPS
7	Rest or 30 mins walk/ yoga	90 mins easy pace on muddy, hilly trails, 6 strides to finish	60 mins easy pace on easy trails	15 mins warm-up jog easy pace, 4 x 4-min hill reps very hard effort, 15 mins easy jog back	Rest or 30 mins walk/ yoga	Warm up 5 mins, 60 mins strength work, cool down 5 mins. Warm up 10 mins, tempo run 20 mins or 5k race, such as parkrun	3 hrs 30 mins easy pace on similar trails to your chosen race	Gather the support of friends, and if running for charity, shout about it even more
8	Rest or 30 mins walk/ yoga	90 mins easy pace on muddy, hilly trails, 6 strides to finish	60 mins easy pace on easy trails	15 mins warm-up jog easy pace, 15 mins tempo run hard effort, 15 mins easy jog back	Rest or 30 mins walk/ yoga	Warm up 5 mins, 30 mins strength work, cool down 5 mins. Easy run 30 mins	2 hrs easy pace on similar trails to your chosen race	EASY WEEK Concentrate on good form, posture, technique and breathing and continue this through to the race
9	Rest or 30 mins walk/ yoga	90 mins easy pace on muddy, hilly trails, 6 strides to finish	60 mins easy pace on easy trails	15 mins warm-up jog easy pace, 5 x 4-min hill reps very hard effort, 15 mins easy jog back	Rest or 30 mins walk/ yoga	Warm up 5 mins, 60 mins strength work, cool down 5 mins. Easy run 60 mins	Half marathon trail race	PEAK WEEK Pick a half marathon race with similar terrain to your race. Reflect on race strategy afterwards
10	Rest or 30 mins walk/ yoga	90 mins easy pace on muddy, hilly trails, 6 strides to finish	60 mins easy pace on easy trails	15 mins warm-up jog easy pace, 30 mins tempo run hard effort, 15 mins easy jog back	Rest or 30 mins walk/ yoga	Warm up 5 mins, 60 mins strength work, cool down 5 mins. Easy run 60 mins	3 hrs easy pace on similar trails to your chosen race	Run in the gear you want to race in to make sure it doesn't chafe and check the mandatory kit list, to avoid last-minute stress
11	Rest or 30 mins walk/ yoga	60 mins easy pace on muddy, hilly trails, 6 strides to finish	60 mins easy pace on easy trails	15 mins warm-up jog easy pace, 6 x 90-sec hill reps very hard effort, 15 mins easy jog back	Rest or 30 mins walk/ yoga	Warm up 5 mins, 30 mins strength work, cool down 5 mins. Easy run 30 mins	2 hrs easy pace on gently hilly trails	EASY WEEK Eat healthily, stay well hydrated and get enough sleep this week and imagine sprinting over the finish line
12	Rest or 30 mins walk/ yoga	60 mins easy pace on muddy trails with gentle hills, 6 strides to finish	Rest or 30 mins walk/ yoga	60 mins easy pace on muddy trails with gentle hills	Rest or 30 mins walk/ yoga	Rest or 30 mins walk/ yoga	Marathon trail run or race!	Take it very easy in preparation for your best marathon ever

WEEK	MON REST	TUES TEMPO	WEDS REST	THURS HILL REPS/ TEMPO RUN	FRI REST	SAT STRENGTH & RUN	SUN LONG RUN	MOTIVATION
9A	Rest or 30 mins walk/ yoga	90 mins easy pace on muddy, hilly trails, 6 strides to finish	60 mins easy pace with gentle hills	15 mins warm-up jog easy pace, 15 mins tempo run hard effort, 15 mins easy jog back	Rest or 30 mins walk/ yoga	Warm up 5 mins, 60 mins strength work, cool down 5 mins. Easy run 60 mins	2 hrs easy pace on similar trails to your chosen race	EASY WEEK Experiment with different nutrition now rather than during the race
9B	Rest or 30 mins walk/ yoga	90 mins easy pace on muddy, hilly trails, 6 strides to finish	60 mins easy pace with gentle hills	15 mins warm-up jog easy pace, 6 x 3-min hill reps very hard effort, 15 mins easy jog back	Rest or 30 mins walk/ yoga	Warm up 5 mins, 60 mins strength work, cool down 5 mins. Easy run 60 mins	3 hrs easy pace on similar trails to your chosen race	Check your gear fits well and doesn't chafe on these longer distances
9C	Rest or 30 mins walk/ yoga	90 mins easy pace on muddy, hilly trails, 6 strides to finish	60 mins easy pace with gentle hills	15 mins warm-up jog easy pace, 15 mins tempo run hard effort, 15 mins easy jog back	Rest or 30 mins walk/ yoga	Warm up 5 mins, 60 mins strength work, cool down 5 mins. Easy run 60 mins	Trail marathon	PEAK WEEK Set off slower than you think you should and practise speed hiking steep, long hills

TRAIL HACK

AVOID BURN-OUT

A few weeks contain two fast sessions, such as hill reps or a tempo run, and a parkrun or half marathon. If you feel overly fatigued or on the edge of an injury, exchange one of these fast sessions for an easy run or cross-training, to recover.

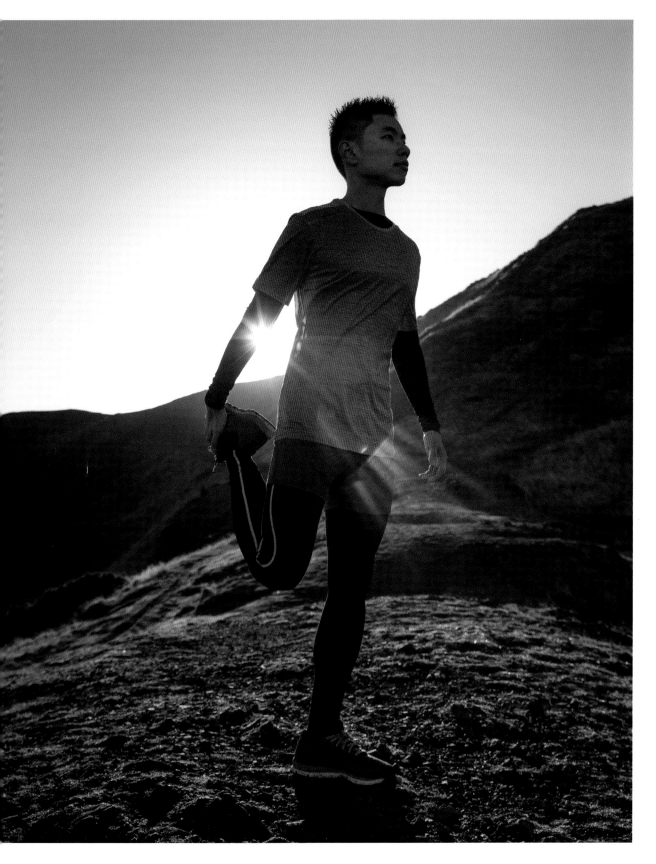

4

BEAT INJURY

Injury is sadly a part of so many people's running journey, especially if you get properly bitten by the bug and run too far or too often too soon. This chapter will help you avoid injury altogether, nip it in the bud quicker, or cure the most common complaints.

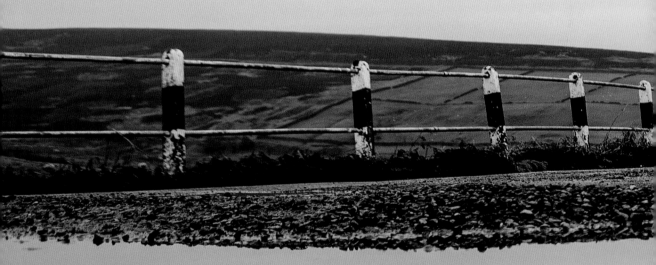

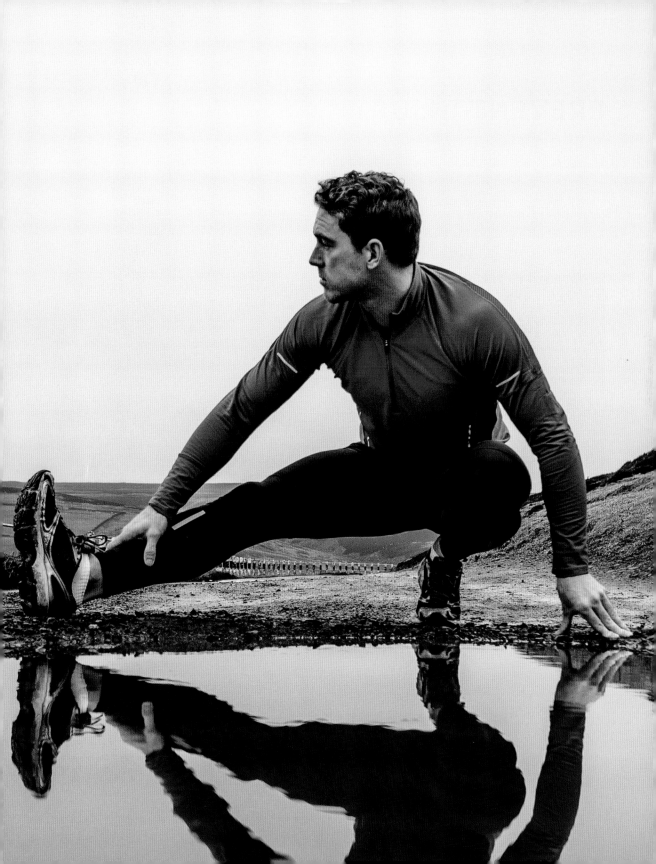

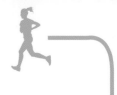

PREVENT INJURY

If you want to run throughout your whole life, look after your body like the prized possession it truly is. Follow this simple but effective guidance for faster recovery and injury prevention.

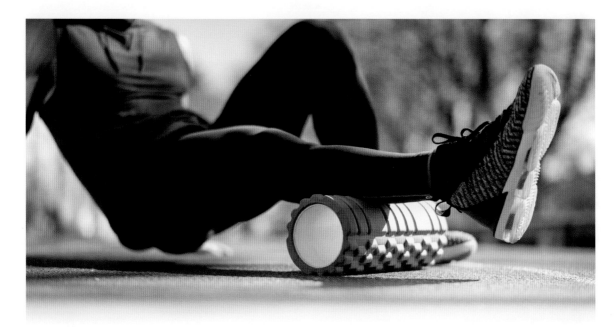

1 SLEEP WELL

Good sleep is vital for your body's repair process. Aim for 8 hours a night, and practise good sleep hygiene – avoid large meals late at night, avoid bright lights 1–2 hours before bed, take a relaxing bath, prepare your bedroom for a peaceful night with a cool temperature.

2 EAT WELL

Eat lots of different-coloured fruit and veg (especially dark, leafy greens) for plenty of nutrients and minerals, along with protein-rich lean meat, pulses, beans and carbs, such as sweet potato and brown rice, which help with repair.

3 REST WELL

Your body needs time to recover and rebuild stronger and if you don't rest it will break down and become injured. Sandwich intense or long sessions with rest days or active recovery such as walking.

4 STRETCH MORE

Think about the time you spend on social media or watching the TV. Maybe it isn't too hard to fit in stretching every day after all? Turn to pp. 63–65 for the best moves.

5 STRENGTHEN

Unless you have a physical job, sitting at a desk all day switches off your glutes (bum muscles), does nothing to engage your core muscles, and shortens your hamstrings (backs of your legs), so follow the prehab moves on pp. 124–126 and strength workout on p. 66 to make sure your body is as strong as possible for running.

6 CROSS-TRAIN

Doing exercise other than running uses different muscle groups, which is great for preventing overuse injuries, and if it's lower impact than running – such as swimming and cycling – it helps you keep fit without putting the same stress on your joints.

7 BE AWARE OF OVERTRAINING

Overtraining can be difficult to spot as you need to stress your body in order to improve, which means you may think that feeling tired is normal. However, if you feel fatigued with sore muscles that don't recover after a few days, you might be overdoing it. Other signs include performance that might have plateaued or worsened, you might feel lethargic all the time, your mojo might have gone, you might feel irritable or depressed, you might be gaining weight, getting ill a lot and your resting heart rate might be higher by 7–10 beats per minute. If you ignore these symptoms, overtraining can get worse, but if you take a few days' rest and lighten your training volume and/or intensity, these effects can be reversed quickly.

8 SEEK HELP EARLY ON

Have you ever met a runner who has ignored their injury, not sought professional advice and simply run on until it was too painful to continue? We all get the odd ache or pain when we run, but if something persistently bothers you, or a clear injury happens, do visit a trusted local sports professional rather than take your symptoms to the internet. What helped someone else might even be harmful to you, so get a diagnosis from an expert and do all the exercises they give you.

9 HAVE A REGULAR PHYSIO SESSION

Yes, this does add up financially, but rather than buying new gear or entering a race, invest in your body first or you may not be able to make use of either of those things. Seeing a physio once a month for a check-up and sports massage is a fantastic way to stop injuries in their tracks and highlight weak areas for strengthening.

TRAINING DURING ILLNESS

It's not a good idea to run while you're ill because your body needs to put its energies into getting you back to 100 per cent. Easy exercise such as walking, yoga and stretching is fine if you're going stir crazy, but intense exercise like running will overstretch your already hard-working immune system and prolong your illness, even if it's just a sore throat, cold or runny nose. Eat healthily, rest, and you will recover faster. Go easy on your first week back into running to be sure your illness is totally over, then it's back to normal.

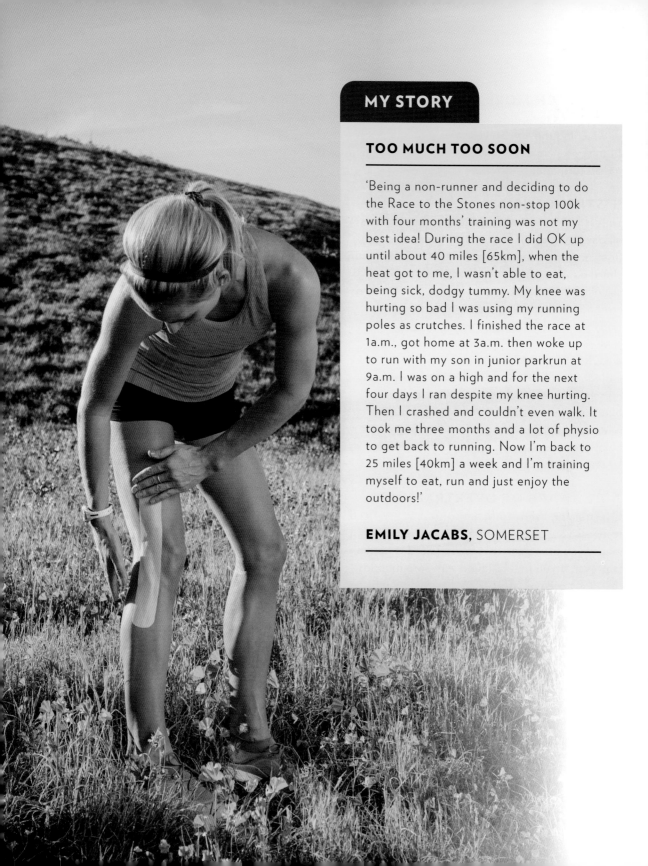

TOO MUCH TOO SOON

'Being a non-runner and deciding to do the Race to the Stones non-stop 100k with four months' training was not my best idea! During the race I did OK up until about 40 miles [65km], when the heat got to me, I wasn't able to eat, being sick, dodgy tummy. My knee was hurting so bad I was using my running poles as crutches. I finished the race at 1a.m., got home at 3a.m. then woke up to run with my son in junior parkrun at 9a.m. I was on a high and for the next four days I ran despite my knee hurting. Then I crashed and couldn't even walk. It took me three months and a lot of physio to get back to running. Now I'm back to 25 miles [40km] a week and I'm training myself to eat, run and just enjoy the outdoors!'

EMILY JACABS, SOMERSET

COMMON INJURIES

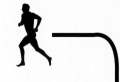

Have you ever met an experienced runner who has never had an injury? They're a rare breed as running is such a high-impact sport. What's more, such a lot of us simply like to run and struggle to get motivated for strength work. Here are the most common injuries and how to avoid or rehab them.

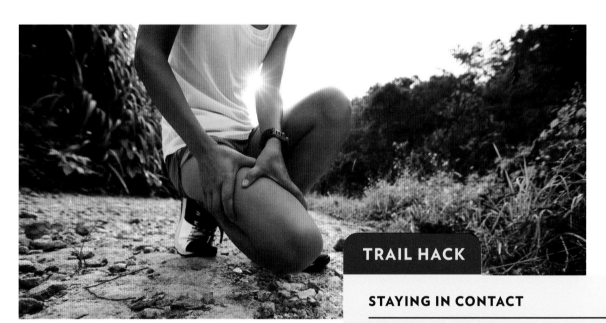

TRAIL HACK

STAYING IN CONTACT

Coping with injury is tough, especially if your running club is also your social life. So don't miss out on the craic – in the past I have cycled to meet my club before they ran, then did a cycle or swim during their run and rejoined them for the chat at the end too. You could also use the extra time to pursue an entirely different hobby for a while, such as joining a choir or life-drawing class.

MEET THE EXPERT

The information on the most common injuries and the prehab moves in this section is from renowned sports physio Paul Hobrough, who has worked with record-breaking Olympic runners Steve Cram and Paula Radcliffe as well as regular running clients. His book, *Running Free of Injuries*, is your ultimate source of information for sorting out niggles fast and curing injuries quickly. https://physioandtherapy.co.uk

INJURY POSITIVITY

'I tried everything for my bunions – K-tape, orthotics, bunion pads, wider shoes, cutting holes in my shoes and physio strength exercises. But the pain got so bad I needed surgery, with three months' recovery. I squeezed in my first ultra before the op in case things didn't go well, and started daily meditation and a gratitude journal. Post op, I volunteered at parkrun in my wheelchair, did strength exercises, watched inspiring running films, kept in touch with club friends and joined a bunion surgery support group. I'm trying to be positive and concentrate on the things I can do. It's hard, there have been tears, but it makes you more mentally resilient in the long run (pun intended), which is great training for trail running.'

KATE SHEPHARD, NEAR BIRMINGHAM

FOOT PAIN

The foot is a wonderfully intricate piece of machinery and there are quite a few injuries that can occur in this area. One of the most common is plantar fasciitis – inflammation to the connective tissue along the sole of the foot. It can often strike those who stand for long periods, such as the old 'bobby on the beat' who gave it its colloquial name: 'policeman's heel'.

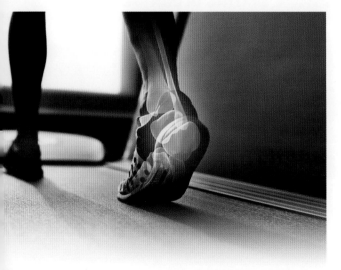

SYMPTOMS

Sharp pain on the inside of the heel, feeling like you're standing on a stone in the morning, pain that wears off after a few steps and eases for the rest of the day, pain again after you've been off your feet for a while.

CURE IT

Treatment is very varied and there is evidence to show that some sufferers can benefit from shockwave therapy if the following don't work:

- Wear insoles to support your arch.
- Don't walk barefoot, even round the house.
- Stretch your calf (both muscles, see p. 63).
- Write the alphabet with your foot in the air before moving after any significant period of rest.
- Ice the foot after a long time standing or walking.
- Get calf and foot massages.

- Wear a plantar fasciitis sock to keep a mild stretch on the connective tissue overnight.
- Use anti-inflammatory medication if you can without side-effects (see your GP for direction).

GET RUNNING AGAIN

You need to return gradually so as not to overload the fascia and prolong the injury. Do short, three-minute rehab runs then stretch both calf muscles (see p. 63). Do 5 repetitions if there is no pain. Rest for two days, then repeat. After two pain-free weeks, you can start to increase the rehab runs by one minute, reducing the number of repetitions as your runs get longer.

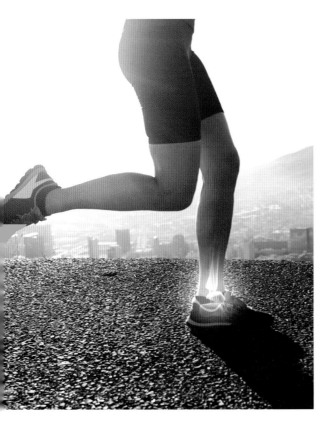

ANKLE SPRAIN

Surprisingly, many trail runners report spraining an ankle while on easy ground rather than negotiating difficult rocky or tussocky terrain! This could be due to a lack of focus once the 'danger' is passed, so remind yourself to pay attention to the ground at all times, however easy it may seem.

SYMPTOMS

Sudden acute pain at the ankle (usually the outer side) while turning, landing or slipping awkwardly, immediate swelling at the ankle. In severe cases you will not be able to put any weight on the affected leg.

CURE IT

Your body is already repairing your ankle during the first four-day inflammatory phase, so avoid using anti-inflammatory medicine, which will inhibit this healing process, and only use ice, compression and elevation if you are still in a great deal of pain, even at rest. After three days, get a massage from a qualified sports physio and begin strengthening and balance exercises (*see* p. 66) if possible.

GET RUNNING AGAIN

This depends on the severity of the sprain, but if it's severe, it may take six–eight weeks, or even surgery if you have ruptured a ligament. Build up very gradually with a few miles at a time, on easy ground at first, concentrating on foot placement. Do strengthening exercises at least a couple of hours before running so you don't exhaust your key stabilising muscles just before you need to use them.

ACHILLES PAIN

This is one of the most common injuries in runners. The Achilles is a tendon that attaches your calf muscles to your heel bone and it can become stiff, tight and eventually too painful to run through. It's important to get this injury checked out before it becomes chronic and difficult to shift.

SYMPTOMS

Pain at the back of the heel, tight calf muscles, difficulty lifting the toes up, and a painful and stiff calf and Achilles for the first few steps in the morning.

CURE IT

Your physio should give you regular massage, especially to the calf, ankle and foot area, and they may also suggest shockwave therapy in severe cases. Most will be solved with gradual strengthening, from calf raises and lowers, building up to holding a weight or wearing a weighted backpack.

GET RUNNING AGAIN

Build up gradually, mile by mile, only running if the pain isn't more than uncomfortable at any time during the run.

SHIN SPLINTS

This is the layman's term for medial tibial stress syndrome, which particularly affects new runners or runners who have significantly upped their training volume or intensity over a short period of time. It can be due to poor biomechanics or overtraining.

SYMPTOMS

Tightening of the calf muscles, dull aching at the front of the lower leg (in the shin area), pain at the start and end of the run, worsening pain during the run, pain even when walking, pain lifting the toes against resistance, difficulty pointing the toes.

CURE IT

The muscle does not become stronger just by fighting through the pain, so you must stop running until the pain eases and start cross-training with activities that don't aggravate the area. Speed up recovery by icing and stretching the shins, stretch the calf muscles and get a lower leg massage.

GET RUNNING AGAIN

Run on soft surfaces where possible (aqua-jogging and treadmills also provide some impact relief here) and run for three minutes, then stretch the calf muscles, then do 4 more repetitions until you can run pain-free. Then up the minutes run and lower the number of repetitions as you recover.

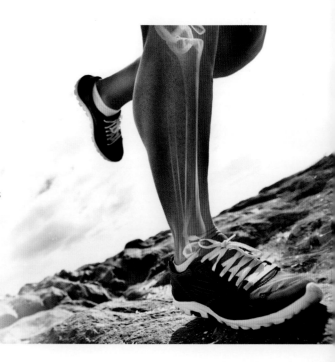

KNEE PAIN

There are many reasons why you may get knee pain, but one of the most common afflictions is runner's knee (patellofemoral pain syndrome, PFPS). This is closely linked to ITB pain (see next column), and is a wear-and-tear injury caused by friction between the kneecap (patella) and base of the thigh bone (femur).

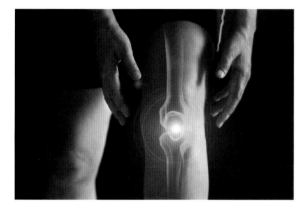

SYMPTOMS
Pain behind the kneecap when it is pressed or during running, especially downhill, pain walking down stairs, pain when performing a single-legged squat on the injured side.

CURE IT
You need to stretch and strengthen up your glutes (bum muscles) and hip flexors, and work on ankle and core strength. Check out the prehab moves on pp. 124–126 to work on these areas. Have a gait analysis to see why the problem occurs in the first place and work on the weaknesses that are found. Kinesiology tape (K-tape) can also help (see pp. 130–131).

GET BACK TO RUNNING
Tape the knee to allow you to run while you continue with your strength exercises (don't do them just before running as this will fatigue them). Then say bye to the tape once your muscles are strong enough to support you without pain. Keep up the strength exercises though – they should form part of your weekly routine now.

ITB PAIN

Iliotibial band (ITB) syndrome is one of the most common running injuries and often co-exists or gets confused with runner's knee (see Knee Pain). Your ITB is a super-strong band running from the outside of your hip to the outside of your knee and it helps keep your knee aligned. Pain comes from friction at the knee joint due to the tightening of the two muscles that hold it in place: the gluteus maximus (your largest bum muscle) and the tensor fascia latae (TFL) at your hip.

SYMPTOMS
Pain at the outside of the knee while running that stops when you stop running, pain going downhill but not uphill, pain worsening as you continue running, until you stop.

CURE IT
The ITB itself cannot be stretched or lengthened so the key is to release the tight muscles controlling this band, then strengthen the rest of the body to support the natural functioning of the ITB. It's a good idea to have a gait analysis to work out why this has happened so you can get individual prescription of exercises (such as the prehab moves on pp. 124–126) to strengthen your specific weaknesses and stop further pain. Kinesiology tape (K-tape) can also help; get your physio to show you how to use it, or *see* pp. 130–131.

GET BACK TO RUNNING

You may be able to run pain-free using K-tape while you continue to do your strength exercises (don't do them just before going for a run or you'll tire them out). You can remove the tape once your muscles are strong enough to support you themselves. Keep doing the strengthening exercises or the injury may rear its ugly head again.

DOMS

Although not specifically an injury, it's worth talking about delayed onset muscle soreness (DOMS) here because it can be extremely painful. It is the scourge of the trail runner, especially after hammering down a lot of steep hills when your four thigh muscles (quads) work hard to stabilise you. If you're not used to it or you're racing hard, it overloads the muscle, causing micro-tears and pain. If you refuel and rest right and then keep subjecting yourself to similar and harder downhills your body will repair those micro-tears and become stronger.

SYMPTOMS

Pain in the thighs peaking 24 hours after your run, ranging from mild to so agonising you have to walk or crawl downstairs backwards. Walking on the flat or uphill is usually fine. Pain eases after a couple of days.

CURE IT

There isn't really any cure for DOMS apart from adequate training of the quad muscles to cope with long, steep descents, but even elite athletes can experience DOMS if they push themselves hard on a hilly course. Some experience relief from immersing the thighs for 5–10 minutes in

EXPERT TIP

HOW TO AVOID WEIGHT GAIN WHILE INJURED

'This can be tricky, as if you're not able to keep up the same level of exercise through cross-training, you are likely to gain weight if you eat the same amount, so listen to your body and try not to overeat. Use a smaller plate and eat slowly to give your brain the 10–15 minutes it needs to realise you're full. Eat filling, nutritious foods like veg, fruit and nuts rather than processed high-sugar and/or high-fat foods like cakes, pastries and crisps.'

ANITA BEAN,
SPORTS NUTRITIONIST

a cool lake, river or bath straight after running. In the days after the run, refuel with the right nutrition (see pp. 27–28) and ease the quads with walking, jogging, swimming, easy cycling, gentle stretching and massaging to increase blood flow and encourage muscular repair.

GET BACK TO RUNNING

After a few days' rest you should be good to run again. The first few minutes might be a little sore, but ease in gently and start with a short, steady run. Include more downhill running in your training if you plan on hammering those downhills more often too...

These can sometimes be so agonising they can even prevent you from walking. The best way to avoid blisters is to have well-fitting socks and trail shoes that you've worn in with short runs first. Even so, when you're out for hours pounding through puddles, grit and mud, blisters can strike however comfy your shoes are.

Q: Should I stop?

A: If you're doing a short race it's OK to put up with a burgeoning blister so as not to lose places or your time, but on longer races where you know you'll be out for hours, taking care of your feet comes first. As soon as you feel a blister starting to form (known as a hot spot), take off your shoe, clean the area and get a blister plaster on to protect it.

Q: Which plasters are best?

A: Normal plasters sometimes don't stick very well, so try dedicated blister plasters, which won't peel off until a few days later. If your blister is huge you might need a second skin-style dressing that you can cut to shape, and if they are between your toes you might find K-tape (see pp. 130–131) works best for sticking well and minimising bulk.

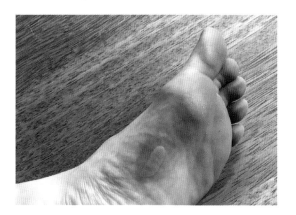

Q: Should I pop it?

A: It's always best to leave the skin unbroken if possible to avoid infection and painful grit getting in, so if your blister is not getting in the way too much or isn't too bulbous, leave it be. However, if the swelling lump of fluid is causing you more pain – for example, if it's between the toes, making them wider and more squashed inside your shoe, you'll want to go for the pop.

Q: How do I pop it?

A: Get a sterile needle (keep one in your first aid kit, see p. 155), or hold a safety pin in a flame for a few seconds to sterilise it, then let it cool. Prick the blister at the base so that the fluid drains with gravity. Gently press it to drain all the fluid and wipe with a sterile wipe, if possible. Dry the area before applying your blister plaster. Hold it down with a warm hand to encourage the glue to stick before you get your sock and shoe back on.

Q: Who can help me?

A: Many races have medics at checkpoints as well as at the start and finish. Other more experienced runners can also guide you and most running clubs will have one or two people with medical backgrounds within their ranks.

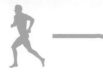

PREHAB EXERCISES

These essential strength moves from sports physio Paul Hobrough, author of *Running Free of Injuries*, will go a long way towards preventing you from getting injured in the first place if you take even five minutes to do two or three moves each day. Combine these with stretches and foam rolling for a well-rounded prehab programme.

FOOT STRENGTH – TOWEL GRABBING

Build arch strength and mobility in the foot by sitting on a chair with a towel spread out in front of it. Put your foot flat on the floor, half on the towel, then grab the towel with your forefoot and scrunch it towards you. Repeat this for two minutes.

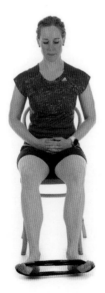

ANKLE STRENGTH – RESISTANCE LOOP

Make a small loop with a resistance band. Sit on a chair, or on the floor with legs straight out in front, and place both feet inside the loop with the band around the forefoot. Push against the band to move the upper foot out to the sides. If it is too easy, move the feet apart a little. Do 3 x 15 repetitions.

TRAIL HACK

TIME IT RIGHT

Perform these in the evening before bed if you can, rather than just before a run, else you risk tiring out the very muscles you are trying to strengthen up for running.

CALF STRENGTH – CALF RAISES

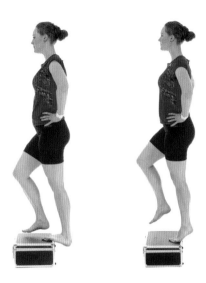

On tiptoes on the edge of a step, lower one foot slowly in a controlled manner until your heel cannot descend any further. Rise on to tiptoes again in a smooth, controlled movement. Do 3 x 15 repetitions, then swap sides.

GLUTE AND HIP STRENGTH – CLAMS

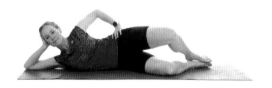

Lie on your side and bend the knees so the soles of your feet are in line with your spine. Slowly lift the top knee up away from the other knee, place a hand on your upper buttock to check the glute is doing the work rather than your leg muscles. Hold for three seconds, then return the knee slowly. Do 3 x 15 repetitions, then swap sides.

CORE STRENGTH – BASIC ACTIVATION TEST

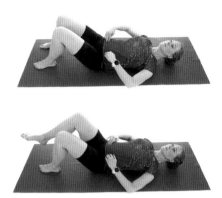

Make sure you're engaging your core properly in all other exercises with this simple activation and strength test. Lie on your back with legs bent at 90 degrees. Find your hip bones poking upwards with both hands, then move your fingers 2.5cm (1in) in and down. Cough and you should feel a muscle bounce under your fingers. If not, move your fingers slightly until you find it. This is the location of your transversus abdominis (TA), part of your core muscles. Imagine you are stopping yourself going for a wee – you should feel the TA tighten. Hold that tension, then draw in your belly button and slightly flatten your lower back towards the floor. Now you are tensing your core muscles accurately.

To test your core for strength, maintain this tension while you lift alternate feet off the floor. Once you can do 25 repetitions on each leg, you are ready to move on to more challenging core exercises.

If you perform the original activation while lying on your front before getting into the plank position you will make sure you are activating the right muscles and may be able to hold the plank for longer and with more ease.

GLUTE ACTIVATION AND CORE STRENGTH – PLANK WITH RAISED LEG

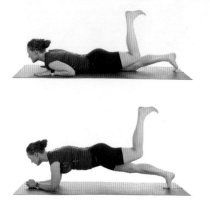

BALANCE AND LEG STRENGTH – SINGLE-LEG BALANCE

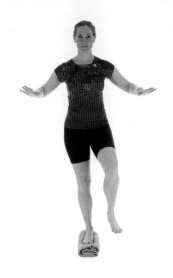

WHOLE-LEG STRENGTH – SINGLE-LEG SQUAT

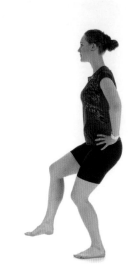

Lie on your front and bend one knee to 90 degrees. Imagine there's a tray of drinks on the sole of the raised foot. Carefully lift the leg upwards using the glute only, taking care not to change the knee bend and spill those drinks! Perform this five times with bent knee, then do five raises with a straight leg. Then swap legs. Make this harder by doing it in a plank position with bent elbows directly under your shoulders, hands clasped together, on tiptoes with legs out straight behind you, stomach muscles engaged.

Stand one-legged on a cushion or rolled-up towel and balance. When you have mastered this and can hold it for 20 seconds, experiment with holding the free leg in a variety of running positions, bringing the knee up and down and moving the arms as if running. Aim to keep your hips level throughout – do it in front of a mirror to check this, if possible. Balance for a total of 60 seconds, then swap legs and repeat.

Stand on one leg with hands on hips. Keep the knee over the middle toe as you stick your bum out, keep your chest up, and lower down as far as you can without the knee moving inwards towards the big toe. Stop if you see this happening and rise up again. Resist the temptation for a deeper squat until you can prevent this inward movement. Start with 10 repetitions on each side, then work on deepening the squat rather than increasing reps.

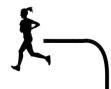

USING A FOAM ROLLER

Studies have linked foam rolling to improved range of motion, flexibility, mobility, reduced muscle soreness, increasing circulation, loosening tight muscles and encouraging stress relief and relaxation. Rolling around on one in front of the TV of an evening is a good way to self-massage and encourage a speedier recovery.

CALVES

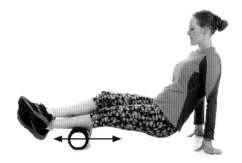

Start off with a calf roll, moving both calves back and forth on the roller, then one at a time with the other foot on the floor.

INCREASE THE INTENSITY
Place one foot on top of the other. Rotate the calf around from left to right to access the whole muscle.

HAMSTRINGS (BACKS OF THE LEGS)

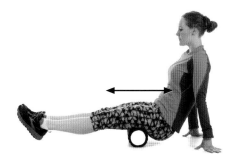

Roll both at the same time, then switch to one and then the other.

INCREASE THE INTENSITY
Place one leg on top of the other to intensify the massage.

GLUTES (BUTTOCKS)

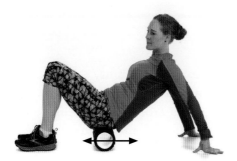

Sit on the roller, roll back and forth and lean to the left and right to access the different glute muscles in this area. Lean to the side and cross one foot over the other knee to access the deep piriformis muscle too.

ITB (OUTSIDE OF THE THIGH)

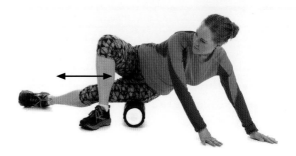

You can't increase the stretch in your ITB (iliotibial band) itself, but it can feel good to lie on your side and roll around the outer knee area and sides of your hips and buttocks to massage the muscles that control it. Support yourself with the upper leg and arm in front of you. Find out more about caring for your ITB on p. 121.

BACK

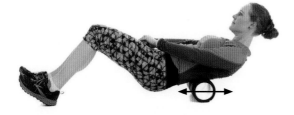

You can play about with this one, using the roller along the knobbles of your spine, across the shoulders, and even edging to one side of the roller to get deeper into the shoulder blades.

TRAIL HACK

FOAM ROLLING DEMO

Want a demonstration of these moves to follow? See my latest foam rolling film in the recovery playlist on Wild Ginger Running YouTube channel.

QUADS (FRONT OF THE THIGH)

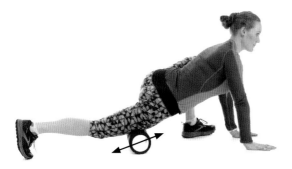

Massage the front of the thighs with arms in a plank position (also good for your core strength). Rock back and forth with the arms as you roll up and down, both thighs together, then do one at a time to intensify the move.

ADDUCTORS (INNER THIGH)

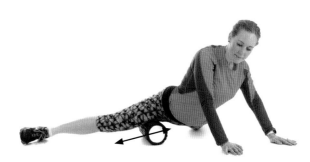

Move to one side of the foam roller to place it under your inner thigh area for a massage to the adductors. With your arms still in the plank position, roll sideways to move your inner thigh back and forth over the roller.

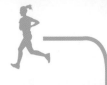

USING K-TAPE

Kinesiology tape (K-tape) is a durable, stretchy elastic tape you can stick to your body to support injured muscles during your rehab programme. It's no substitute for proper rehab, so stick to your prescribed exercises and the prehab moves on pp. 124–126, but it can help you continue running while your body is less than 100 per cent.

See the K-tape demo on Wild Ginger Running YouTube channel for how to do these properly.

ITB (ILIOTIBIAL BAND) SUPPORT

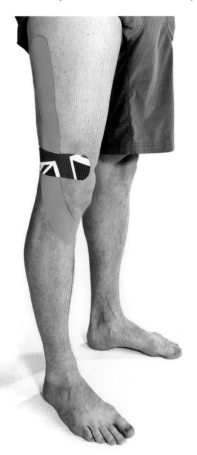

K-TAPE NEEDED
One thigh-length strip and one strip one-third of that length

TAPE IT UP
Stretch out your outer thigh by crossing the affected leg behind the other throughout. Take the longer strip and stick the end on the sore spot on the outside of your knee. Stick the rest of this strip down, applying no stretch to it, all the way up the outside of the thigh in the centre, following the line of the ITB. Then take the shorter strip and tear the paper away in the centre to expose the middle of the tape. Stretch this section about 75 per cent and stick it over the spot where you experience most pain. Then peel the two ends off and stick them down, applying no further stretch.

TRAIL HACK

MAKE IT STICK

Once you've taped yourself up, rub your warm hands all over the tape for a minute or two to activate the glue and make it stick for the whole of your run or race.

KNEE SUPPORT

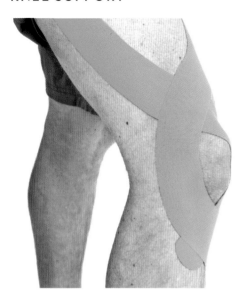

K-TAPE NEEDED
Two strips both the length of your thigh

TAPE IT UP
In a standing position, stick the end of the first strip diagonally under your knee with no stretch to it. Then bend your knee by 90 degrees (you could place it on a chair behind you) and stick the tape around your kneecap with 50 per cent stretch until you reach the centre of your thigh. Continue sticking the rest of the strip down with no stretch on the tape. Repeat on the other side with the second strip.

SHIN SPLINT SUPPORT

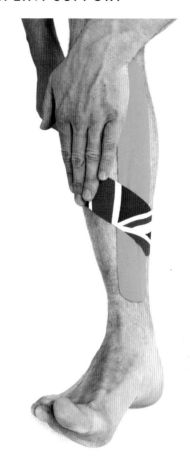

K-TAPE NEEDED
One strip shin-length, one 10cm (4in) strip

TAPE IT UP
Stretch your foot out in front of you with the toes pointing upwards throughout. Stick the longer strip with no stretch along the inside edge of your shin bone. Stick the 10cm (4in) strip across the point of maximum pain, diagonally across the long strip with 75 per cent stretch for the most support.

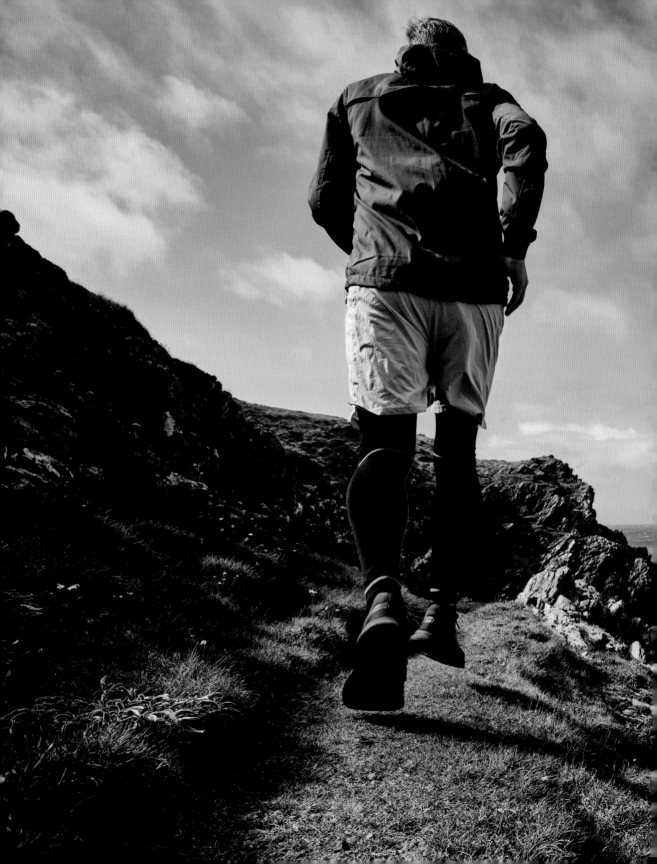

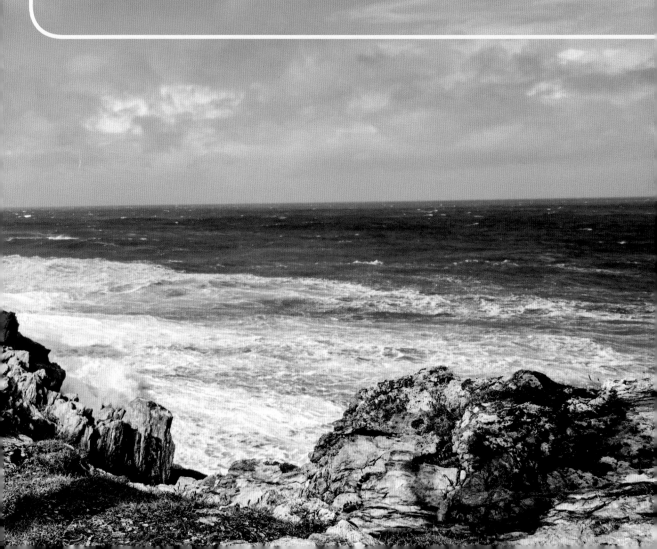

5

TRAIL GEAR

Like all sports, there's an unlimited amount of gear you can empty your wallet on, so here are the main items you might want to consider and what to look for to make sure you make the right purchase the first time round.

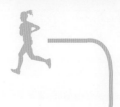

TRAIL SHOES

To start with, if the terrain is not too muddy, uneven and rocky, you can happily use your road running shoes for easy off-road running on canal towpaths, gravel tracks through country parks and well-maintained forest trails. If you're new to running and want to start on these types of trails, a well-fitting pair of road trainers with a bit of grip is a good start. However, if you know you'll be running in more squelchy stuff, head straight for the trail shoes. Once you start to hit the mud, bog and wet grass you'll need a shoe with a lot more grip and possibly less cushioning so you can feel and respond quickly to the uneven ground. Here's what to look for.

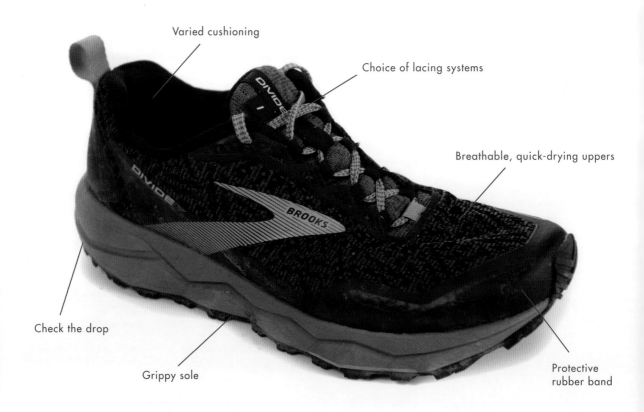

Varied cushioning

Choice of lacing systems

Breathable, quick-drying uppers

Check the drop

Grippy sole

Protective rubber band

GRIP

This is the biggest visible difference between road and trail shoes. Trail shoes have more grip – deeper, more aggressive lugs for traction on mixed terrain, such as squelchy, muddy, grassy, gritty and rocky ground and the odd road section. Trail shoe grip varies from slightly more than road shoes to larger lugs that really bite into the mud. Fell running shoes go all the way, with football stud-like lugs for the gloopiest of off-path mountain running.

DROP

The drop is the height difference between the heel and the toe. Traditional road shoes (not athletics spikes) often have a stacked heel with a 10–12mm drop. Trail shoes are closer to the ground and have less cushioning, to allow you to feel the uneven terrain, often with a 4–8mm drop, sometimes even zero. Check the drop of your current shoes versus any new shoe as a sudden change can strain your calf muscles and Achilles tendon. This can lead to injury if you don't transition slowly enough – over months rather than days. See p. 137 for how to transition safely.

CUSHIONING

This is a very interesting topic, still hotly debated in the trail running community. Some trail shoes have a great deal of cushioning, and some have a similar amount to road shoes. However, more minimalist shoes have less cushioning to allow the foot to feel and respond to the uneven ground and encourage a more natural running style, from the days when humans went barefoot or wore simple sandals. Reduce cushioning only gradually as you become more experienced. See the next pages for more.

SUPPORT

Trail shoes don't usually have the same level of support as road shoes. The idea is that as the ground is so uneven, different muscles fire each time and any attempt by the shoe to always encourage the foot one way or the other would either be in vain or possibly even a hindrance. Many brands also encourage natural foot movement without bolstering it too much within the shoe. You can add insoles or heel pads if you need support.

UPPERS

Trail shoe uppers tend to be tough, with a rubber rand at the front to guard against rocks. They are breathable, allowing water in but also out again, and made of quick-drying fabrics that when combined with a good-quality sports sock dry out as you run. You can get waterproof uppers too, which are good for wind, snow, light rain, wet grass and small puddles on easy ground, but in deeper mud and bog, water goes over the top and can't get out again. For this reason, if you only buy one pair, non-waterproof is best.

LACING

Some trail shoes have a thin, wire-like, pull-cord lacing system, which works brilliantly for many, while others struggle to achieve a snug fit. On some, you can re-thread the shoe

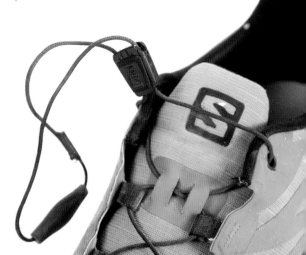

with traditional laces, but some don't have large enough lace holes to do this. Some shoes also have skinnier or rounder laces. The former can cheese-wire your feet and be more fiddly with cold fingers, while the latter can come undone more easily. These laces are more easily swapped out for the best type: slightly stretchy, flattish, wide laces that don't come undone during your run.

MINIMAL AND MAXIMAL SHOES

Trends in running come and go, but over the past decade there have been proponents for both minimal and maximal shoes. The former are low-drop shoes stripped of cushioning, encouraging the foot to work as naturally and efficiently as possible to mimic barefoot running. The latter have more cushioning than usual, with the idea of protecting the foot and leg joints from the pounding of long distance ultra running events, like a full-suspension mountain bike. Obviously, with these two schools of thought being so diametrically opposed it's hard to know which one might be right for you!

My theory is, if it ain't broke, don't fix it. If you are fine in your regular trail running shoes, not getting injured and feel enough of the terrain beneath your feet to respond quickly to the lumps and bumps underfoot, then your shoe choice is already great and it might lead to injury if you change things dramatically. However, if you keep getting the same injury problems or can't feel enough or too much of the terrain beneath your feet, you might want to consider a more minimal or maximal shoe as appropriate.

TRAIL HACK

FIT IS KING!

Fit is the most important feature of any running shoe – no matter how grippy or which elite athlete wears it, you won't be running far if they give you blisters or pinch your toes. That's why it's best to visit your nearest independent running shop to try on as many pairs as possible with advice from staff who are passionate about running.

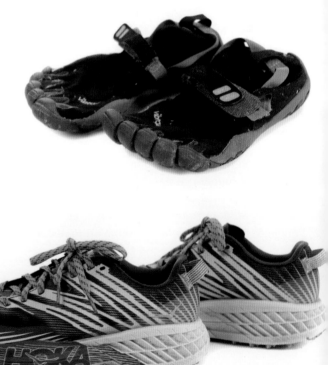

SHOULD YOU WEAR MINIMAL SHOES?

You might have been intrigued by the barefoot movement around the 2010s, especially if you've read Chris McDougall's famous book *Born to Run*, about the incredible running feats of the Mexican Tarahumara Indians in their traditional huaraches (sandals).

It's widely known that humans used to run barefoot or in sandals, and some still do. So you might think 'aha, all humans are born to run barefoot'. However, if you've been walking and running in shoes all your life, your body will not be used to barefoot running and may need longer than you might think to adapt without straining your Achilles tendon and calf muscles. There's also the more sedentary Western lifestyle and overindulgent diet to consider, which results in heavier, weaker bodies that put more force through the unadapted foot and lower leg, which can lead to stress fractures.

Some believe that wearing minimal shoes forces runners to adopt a more natural running style with a front or whole foot plant rather than the common heel strike made possible by padded trainers. However, although this can be the case for some, in many instances it's difficult to change running technique immediately and hard to maintain once fatigued. This can result in runners inadvertently heel striking in minimal shoes, causing more damage and injury. For technique advice see p. 50.

TRANSITION TO MINIMAL SHOES

If you think minimal shoes are the way to go, be sure to transition slowly over months or even years rather than weeks. This is so that your foot and lower leg muscles, tendons and ligaments can get used to the increased stretch to the Achilles and calf that lower-drop shoes cause. If you try to shortcut this process it can result in painful, long-lasting injury.

1. Start with a shoe with 2–4mm lower drop than you're used to, no more than 4mm lower in one shoe shift. It doesn't sound like much but it really does make a difference to the level of strain and stress you put through the lower leg while running.
2. Begin walking around the house whenever you can in the new low-drop shoes, then wear them outside for short errands or walks. Do this until you can walk a few miles or for an hour comfortably in them with no lower-leg strain afterwards.
3. Start light jogging on a soft surface for 5–10 minutes at first. A good way to do this is to pop them in your running pack, jog to a grassy park or field area, then use them for a short while at the start of your run, before changing back to your usual shoes.
4. Gradually increase your mileage in your low-drop shoes. Once you can run your desired distance comfortably, you can start to work on speed in the same way – speeding up for 5–10 minutes at first, then gradually increasing that timeframe.

If you experience any prolonged discomfort in the foot or leg during transitioning, take a step back and hop into your regular shoes for longer. Most people will find they have a limit with low-drop shoes, beyond which they experience niggles and then injury if they don't heed the signs. For some, this can be zero drop, others might find it at 5mm (0.2in). It's very important to listen to your body to avoid getting injured.

BAREFOOT BRITAIN

'In 2019, I ran 2352 miles [3785km] across Britain completely barefoot, from the Shetland Islands via the Channel Islands, finishing in London. It was an idea I'd had for years as I'd already run 2000 miles [3200km] with shoes on across New Zealand, so I wanted to push myself even further and use the journey to speak to young girls about seeking out challenges of their own. It took two years to transition to running barefoot and I did it gradually. I'd run in normal shoes, then do the last few miles in minimalist shoes, then socks, then completely barefoot. Human bodies are amazing and mine coped well, in training and during the run too. The only hold-ups during my six-month adventure were an infected foot after I cut it on glass, and tonsillitis. All in all – pretty good!'

ANNA MCNUFF, ADVENTURER, AUTHOR AND SPEAKER

SHOULD YOU WEAR MAXIMAL SHOES?

On the other side of the coin, some runners find maximal, highly cushioned shoes help on long-distance ultramarathons and recovery runs after long-distance events. I've also spoken to heavier runners and runners with knee and leg joint problems who have benefited from the increased cushioning on impact. However, I've also met others who are convinced that this cushioning increased the strain on their knee joints and dampened their body's natural ability to absorb impact. So again, as with the minimal shoes, proceed with caution as everyone has different needs.

NOTE THE DROP

One other element can confuse with maximal shoes and that's the drop. With such a large amount of cushioning, it is sometimes overlooked that maximal shoes can also be zero drop. Remember, drop is the height difference between heel and toe, nothing to do with how high the whole shoe is off the ground. So when choosing a shoe with more cushioning but also with a lower drop than you are used to, transition gradually to avoid the chance of injury, following the steps on p. 137.

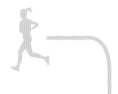

RUNNING CLOTHING

You can spend your entire year's wages on the lightest, most technical new kit, but you can also start off with your old cotton T-shirt, hoodie and joggers and gradually upgrade your wardrobe. The only exception to this is a sports bra – never scrimp on this important bit of kit if you're a woman – to avoid the pain and damage of excessive bounce.

SOCKS

Socks play a major role in preventing blisters for any kind of running, but on trails your foot is more likely to be sliding all over the place so it's vital to get a snug, elasticated fit. Depending on what creates the best fit for your foot in your shoes, you can choose from very thin and breathable to very padded, warm socks. Double-layer socks can also help prevent blisters. Look for natural anti-odour and quick-drying yarn blends such as merino wool, bamboo and moisture-wicking fabrics, such as Coolmax®. Socks that come above the ankle are best so you can easily pull them back up if they slip down, and if you clip your ankle with the other foot as you run, it doesn't hurt as much.

SPORTS BRA

One of the most important bits of kit for women. You might need a different size to your non-running bra, so try plenty of different designs, and jump and jog around the shop to check your bra is definitely beating the bounce.

PANTS

Treat yourself to a couple of pairs of quick-drying, seamless, chafe-free undies and you'll thank yourself on longer, wetter runs!

SHORTS/ TIGHTS

There are so many options now, from simple tight shorts to twin-skin shorts for men, which are tight around the legs but have free-flowing shorts around them for modesty, to shorts with skirts over the top (skorts) for women. Leggings range from three-quarters to full-length and you can find lots of amazing bright, funky patterns now. Rubber rims at the knee or ankle can help prevent ride up but may rub some people. Look for zips at the ankle of full-length leggings, a waist drawcord and a zip pocket big enough for your phone at the back.

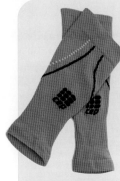

COMPRESSION CLOTHING – DOES IT WORK?

Compression tights, calf guards and long socks are popular with some runners, while others avoid them at all costs. Here's the science...

T-SHIRT OR LONG-SLEEVED TOP

Go for a light, technical, fast-drying, moisture-wicking fabric for comfort. Look for flat seams that won't rub if you wear a running pack. Choose between long- or short-sleeved depending on temperature – if in doubt, go long and roll up the sleeves. A quarter-zip at the front is useful for increased ventilation and getting the top on easily. A collar is handy for wearing with a pack as it protects your neck from rubbing, and it also provides more sun protection. On tight-fitting tops, zipped or elasticated pockets for fuel and small bits of kit can be handy too.

POSSIBLY?

The jury is still out as to whether compression clothing boosts performance during running and you should bear in mind that positive research is often funded by compression companies. However, even if it's just a placebo effect, some may enjoy the springy supportive feeling it gives their legs, a reduction in chafing, less muscular vibration and fewer strains or micro muscle fibre damage as the tight fabric holds everything down. Others might feel trapped and hindered by the snug fit, especially once they get warmer.

DEFINITELY

By contrast, there's plenty of scientific research to prove that compression wear improves recovery as it is used medically in the treatment of circulatory diseases. It works by placing pressure on blood vessels, which reduces their diameter and improves blood flow and valve function. This can help increase lactate removal and repair muscles more quickly, and reduce swelling, inflammation and delayed onset muscle soreness (DOMS). They're very useful if you have to sit for a long period after running, such as during a drive home from a race.

TRAIL HACK

WATERPROOF SOCKS

Waterproof socks are also a good option for very muddy, wet trails; combining these with a non-waterproof shoe makes for much warmer feet, especially in cold, windy and wet weather. Your feet may not stay totally dry due to unavoidable sweating, but at worst you'll be warm.

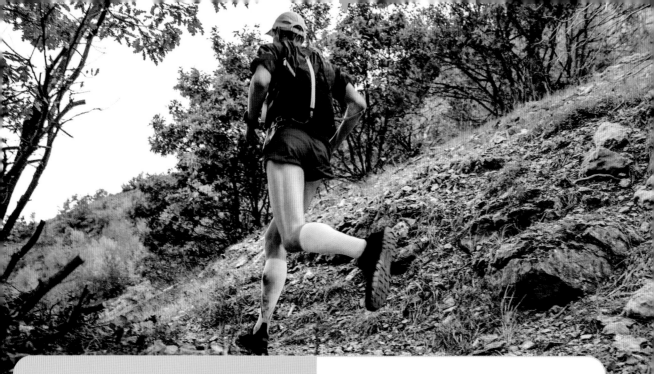

YOUR OPINIONS – COMPRESSION: YES OR NO?

'Love them, either as compression in cold weather or to use as recovery after long, tough runs. I even chop the feet off when they start wearing out on the soles and use them as calf guards!'

Michael Exton, Sheffield

'Not for me – I want to feel the elements on my legs. The freezing cold water, the thick, gloopy mud and the wisp of fern. I want the bramble scratches and the mud stains as a personal trophy – better than any medal or T-shirt.'

Richard Wright, Northamptonshire

'I can't run with them but compression calf sleeves are a definite must after a fell race to help the legs recover."

Don Powell, Basingstoke

'Absolutely love them. Any runs over 10k they are a must for me. Great for trail running, not great for dodgy tans lines in the Sahara...'

Emma Sowden, Stamford

RUNNING JACKETS

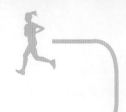

There are quite a few different types of running jacket that are useful in different situations. Here are all the options.

WATERPROOF JACKETS

These can be anything from a super-light and packable emergency layer that you aren't planning to need or use for long, with a simple elasticated hood, cuffs and waist, without pockets, to a full-on, almost hiking/mountaineering jacket, heavier and more protective for remote, all-day mountain running. The latter have more features, such as a fully stormproof, adjustable hood, zip pockets and an adjustable drawcord hem and Velcro cuffs. Choose wisely depending on the forecast, length and remoteness of your run; if in doubt, go for the more protective option every time, for safety.

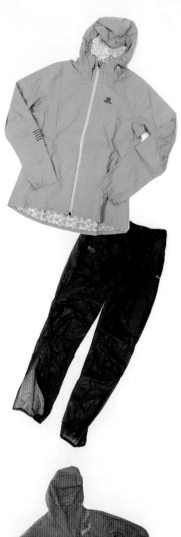

WATERPROOF TROUSERS

While we're on the subject of waterproofs, for waterproof trousers, look for a relaxed fit (not tight to the skin), stretchy fabric, articulated knees (more fabric over the knee area, to allow you complete freedom of movement) and a zip or flare at the ankle so you can put these on easily over your shoes. Pack them unzipped or flared out so you can put them on quickly with minimal faff when the rain starts or the wind picks up.

WINDPROOF JACKET

Also known as wind-resistant or water-resistant jackets, I run more often in a super-light windproof over my T-shirt or long-sleeved top than in any other combination of clothing. The extra warmth this type of jacket gives by cutting out the wind is incredible in relation to its weight and pack size. It will keep off a light shower and drizzle, but it is not waterproof. It's so easy to take off and tie it round your waist or scrunch it in your fist and stuff it in a running pack pocket. If it rains, you can pop your much less breathable waterproof on top and the windproof acts like a slim insulating mid-layer.

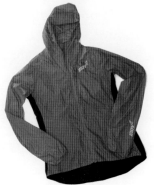

GILET

These can be thermal and/or windproof and insulate your core from the elements, but remember, they have no arms so if you want to take one off, you can't tie it around your waist…

2-IN-1 JACKET

These are rare, but some jackets have zip-off arms so you can use them as a gilet or jacket. Just don't lose those arms!

SYNTHETIC JACKET

Especially on longer or more remote trail runs, it's a great idea to get into the habit of stuffing a super-light, synthetic-fibre insulating jacket in your running pack in case the weather turns or you need to slow down or stop, for injury, fatigue, helping another runner, view-appreciation breaks, wildlife spotting or meeting someone to chat to!

DOWN JACKET

A huge, warm puffer jacket is like putting on your own personal radiator after a long, challenging trail run, especially in winter or wild weather. I

leave mine in the car to grab as soon as I've finished. If you take a down jacket on the run, be aware that down feathers provide less warmth than synthetic insulation if they get wet, so store it in a small dry bag.

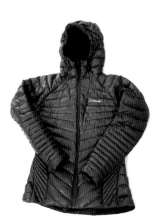

TRAIL HACK

GO LARGE!

Consider buying a waterproof one size too big – it means you can fit your insulating layer underneath and you can quickly throw it on over your running pack for on-and-off showers. This genius manoeuvre avoids too much faffing, stopping, losing time and getting cold.

WHAT ARE TAPED SEAMS?

Mandatory kit lists for races always specify waterproof jackets and trousers (also known as full body cover) with 'fully taped seams'. This is because however waterproof the fabric, sewing the jacket together creates tiny stitch-holes, large enough for rain to seep in. Taping over the seams seals over the stitches to make your jacket or trousers fully waterproof. Windproof, wind-resistant or water-resistant jackets are not fully waterproof because despite being made of highly water-resistant fabrics, the seams are not taped. Just to confuse matters, a waterproof jacket will also be windproof by its very nature, but it's called a waterproof to show its highest level of weather protection. So, waterproofs are not just useful in the rain – use them in windy weather for extra warmth too.

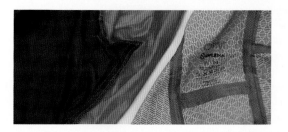

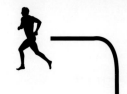

RUNNING PACK VS BUMBAG

Running on uneven, hilly trails with whatever the weather decides to throw at you means distances take longer than they do on roads and you're often in more remote locations with less access to immediate support. A well-designed running pack or bumbag will allow you to carry water, food, kit and first aid without it all bouncing around. Better still, with plenty of easily accessible pockets up front, you can eat, drink and change up your kit on the move. The question is, should you carry it round the waist or on your back?

RUNNING PACK

Larger running packs or race vests can carry more kit. Some find a backpack much comfier than a waistpack, but others can't bear the sweaty back and upper body restriction, however well the pack fits.

FIT

This is the most important aspect to get right to avoid exasperating bounce and chafing. Packs come in specific sizes, women's fit and/or feature adjustment dials and straps that can be used to keep them snug. Shop in your running gear, fill the pack with your intended kit, try it on and jog round the shop to make sure you get the right size.

STYLE

Running packs vary from quite like traditional hiking packs to neat waistcoat-style race vests with loads of pockets up front and easily accessible ones at the side (my preferred option up to 12-litre capacity).

CAPACITY

Think about where and when you'll be running as this dictates the amount of fuel and kit you'll need to take to be safe in the hills. Packs with compression straps or clip-on extra compartments are good for variety.

WEIGHT

This depends on the capacity, but for around the 8–10-litre mark, aim for 250–350g (9–12oz) including bottles. Lighter fabrics are not usually as robust as heavier ones so bear this in mind – many of the more serious runners have a racing and training pack accordingly.

WATER

You can carry it on your back in a 1–2-litre (34–68fl oz) hydration bladder, or in a couple of 400–500ml (13^1/$_2$–17fl oz) soft bottles at the chest or lower down at elbow height using tubes to get the water to your mouth. Lower bottles are usually a comfier option for larger-chested ladies. It's easier to refill soft bottles and tell how much water you've drunk.

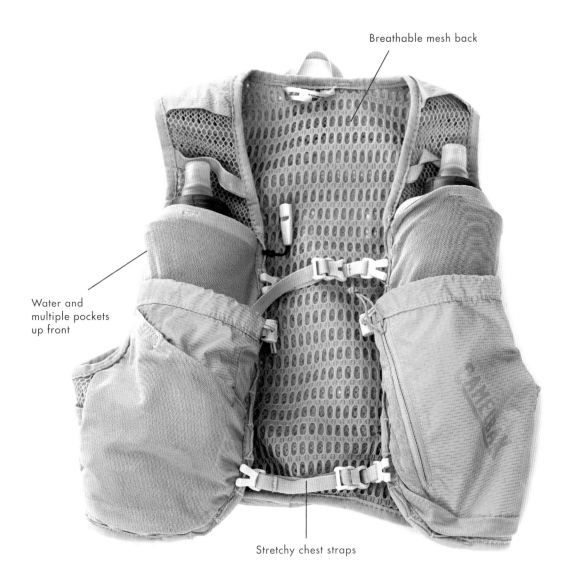

Breathable mesh back

Water and multiple pockets up front

Stretchy chest straps

POCKETS

Look for plenty up front, not obscured by full bottles or drinking tubes. Check your phone fits inside one, at least one zip pocket is great for a key and money, and make sure you can access side pockets without contorting.

POLES

Some packs have dedicated pole attachments down the shoulder straps or across the chest.

Make sure you can access and stow them easily, and that they sit right without irritating you.

EXTRAS

Some have front pouches, back compartments and pole holder quivers that you can retro-fit to the pack. Explore all the options (and whether they bounce!) before you buy.

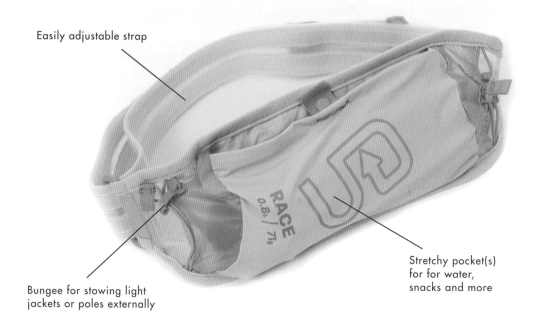

Easily adjustable strap

Bungee for stowing light
jackets or poles externally

Stretchy pocket(s)
for for water,
snacks and more

BUMBAG

Bumbags or waistpacks can't carry as much as
the biggest running packs and they're more often
used for small amounts of kit, with around a
3-litre capacity. Some love the easy, just-spin-it-
round kit access, upper body freedom and sweat-
free back, but others can't get one to stay around
their waist without riding up or bouncing.

FIT AND STYLE

Most have a simple waist adjustment strap, but
you can also get stretchy bands of material with
elastic pockets. For these, you must buy exactly
the right size for your waist.

CAPACITY AND POCKETS

Anything more than 3–4 litres can start to be
cumbersome around the waist, but there are

6-litre waistpacks out there with holsters for
two 500ml (17fl oz) water bottles. At least one
zipped pocket is useful for keys or money.

WEIGHT

The lighter the better with a bumbag – for
example, 120g (5oz) for a simple 3-litre bag.

WATER

The stretchy band design can take a small soft
bottle and some larger bumbags have holsters
for one or two hard plastic bottles. You can get a
lumber hydration bladder for the larger packs too.

POLES

Some bumbags have dedicated pole attachments
using bungee across the main compartment,
which is a fantastic feature.

YOUR OPINIONS

'I prefer a running pack to a bumbag; I find bumbags play havoc with my guts. I always end up needing the loo after running more than a few miles with a bumbag!'

Matt Walker, Gateshead

'I like my 3-litre bumbag for short runs as you can fit everything you need in it and you don't get a sweaty back, especially in the summer.'

Sara Hamblin, Chesterfield

'I mostly use packs but this year tried a waistbelt, which I've really liked for shorter races and runs. Perfect for bars, 500ml [17fl oz] flask and jacket. Also useful on longer runs in combination with a pack.'

Phil Burnett, Dorking

TRAIL HACK

CREATE A FRANKENPACK!

Not got a pocket where you need one? Chop up old gear and sew the pocket on! Seen an extra pack option that doesn't fit on your pack? Sew the attachments on with an old shoelace and hook up your retro-fitted pouches and compartments! Check out the Wild Ginger Running pack reviews playlist on YouTube to choose the right one for you.

RUNNING WATCHES

Once you get more involved in the world of trail running, you might be keen to upgrade from a running app on your phone to a fitness watch that can tell you your heart rate, pace, speed and distance run with ease from your wrist. You can also programme workouts and navigate routes on some more advanced models. Here's a brief run-down of the features to look for.

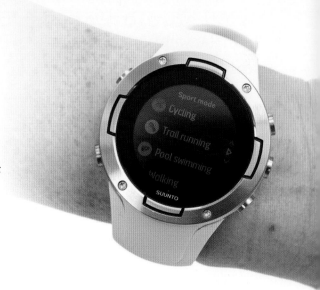

TIME
Sounds silly, doesn't it, but sometimes when a watch is in training mode it's impossible to flick back to see what the actual time is! Make sure that your watch lets you view the real time while in use tracking your run.

BATTERY LIFE
Make sure your watch can keep going as long as you can, or check whether it can continue tracking your run while you charge it with a portable charger.

SPEED AND PACE
Most basic GPS watches will provide this option, and the better ones will also provide pace right now and average pace per split or over the entire run. They may also have a race time predictor for maintenance of a current pace, although this isn't always so useful for trail running as the terrain can vary so much and the hills can confuse the prediction.

HEART RATE
These days, the heart rate (HR) data from the wrist is reliable enough unless you are gunning for peak performance with pinpoint accuracy. I've found especially with mountain running that when your arms and hands get overly cold high on a mountain the wrist sensors can't detect your pulse properly. Even so, I'd recommend a wrist HR over a chest-strap HR monitor because it's much less faff, especially for women also wearing a bra. However, you can also get bras with HR monitor pads in the chest strap, so if you require the utmost in HR accuracy, this may be for you.

INTERVALS
This is a super-useful feature for sessions when you want to work at a certain pace or effort level for a certain amount of time, and then set a rest/recovery time before you repeat this. You can

choose the interval length, the recovery time and the number of repeats you wish to do, and the watch will beep at you when each interval is up so you don't have to keep looking down at it.

NAVIGATION

Navigation on a tiny watch screen can never replace a good old-fashioned map or an app on your phone (as long as you have sufficient battery life and don't get it too wet or drop it), but it is definitely a useful aid and can even be used on its own if the terrain is simple enough. Do be aware of any dangers in following the watch trail exactly though, as it depends how accurately it was created via smartphone or computer, especially when close to cliffs.

ALTITUDE

This is a very useful navigation aid, especially in mountainous areas and in fog, as you can get a reliable reading for how high you are above sea level, which will help you confirm where you are using the contour lines on the map (see p. 56).

MULTI-SPORT OPTIONS

If you're keen on not just running, look for a watch that offers a change of activity profile for sports such as cycling, swimming and gym work, so you can keep track of all your workouts.

SYNCING

Check how your watch syncs up to a program where you can see and analyse your training. Most upload to their own app, but these can vary in their user-friendliness and usefulness. So, many people then have their watch app automatically upload the details to Strava (aka Facebook for sporty people) and analyse it there using the maps, training and gear diary function, pace and heart rate graphs.

OTHER USEFUL FEATURES

CADENCE AND STRIDE LENGTH

Helps you get a feel for whether you are taking the recommended 180 steps per minute, not overstriding and minimising your ground-contact time. However, with trail running, your steps might vary a lot with the terrain and gradient so don't obsess about this.

VIRTUAL COACH

This can be useful as a guide and helps remind you to either run harder or not overdo it based on previous runs, but it doesn't necessarily know what other activities you've been doing and it's not a patch on a real live human being coaching you.

SMART NOTIFICATIONS

If you like to stay in touch rather than escape life while you run, look for watches that sync up with your smartphone to continuously ping you messages and emails on the move.

MUSIC

Many watches now integrate with your smartphone and wireless headphones so you can control music and podcasts on the go.

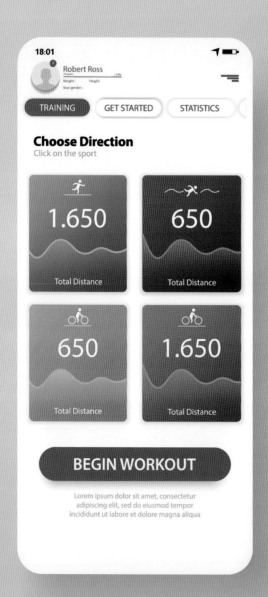

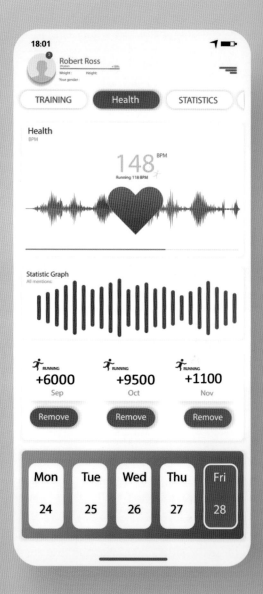

Apps are a great, often free way to plan and log your runs, and to find out interesting training facts, such as how fast you're going and how far you've been. This does mean you have to take your smartphone on the run, so check your leggings pockets are big enough for one, or pop it in your running pack, waistbelt or use an armband.

- **Couch to 5k** – The original get-into-running app from the NHS. Also useful for getting back to running after an injury or time out, with sessions that build you from walk-running to running 5km (3.1 miles) in a couple of months.

- **Zombies Run Game** – Plug your headphones in and listen to one of 200 zombie chasing stories designed to make you speed up, whatever your level.

- **MapMyRun** – A popular run tracker for those who don't have a fitness watch to tell them distance, pace, elevation, calories burned and more.

- **RunKeeper** – Another great run tracker that you can also use to plan and discover routes and create challenges with. It also integrates with Spotify and iTunes playlists.

- **Charity Miles** – Feel even better about your run when you use this app – every time you run with it, you earn money to donate to the charity of your choice.

- **OS Maps** – Extensive UK Ordnance Survey mapping, route planning, GPX file creation on your smartphone and desktop computer; navigation, summit recognition and genius 3D route creation from your phone.

- **ViewRanger** – Global navigation, route planning and tracking app with summit recognition, compatible with Google Earth and health and fitness apps.

- **AllTrails** – Great for the travelling trail runner, this is a global database of trail runs near your location with trail descriptions, trackable routes, distance, elevation and more.

- **Strava** – the Facebook of the fitness world, upload or track your runs, compete with yourself and others on segments, analyse data, write notes, add photos, give kudos to friends and elites. Use global heatmaps to see where others are running most often.

- **TrainingPeaks** – Good for planning your training, since your coach can also plan, view and advise too. Analyses power data if you have a foot pod such as Stryd that attaches to your shoelaces and measures speed, slope, run form, fatigue and wind to deliver perfect pacing advice.

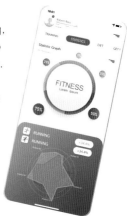

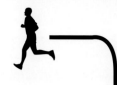

MANDATORY RACE KIT

For your own safety, most trail races have a list of mandatory kit as the minimum that every competitor must take. Always check their website well before the start so you have enough time to borrow or buy anything you don't have, or if you have queries, email the race organiser (RO) before they get too busy before the race. You risk not starting, a time penalty or a disqualification (DQ) if you lack an item. It's a tough job organising a trail race, and it's only with your safety in mind that ROs put together these lists, so do respect them even if you disagree – it's their race and their word is final.

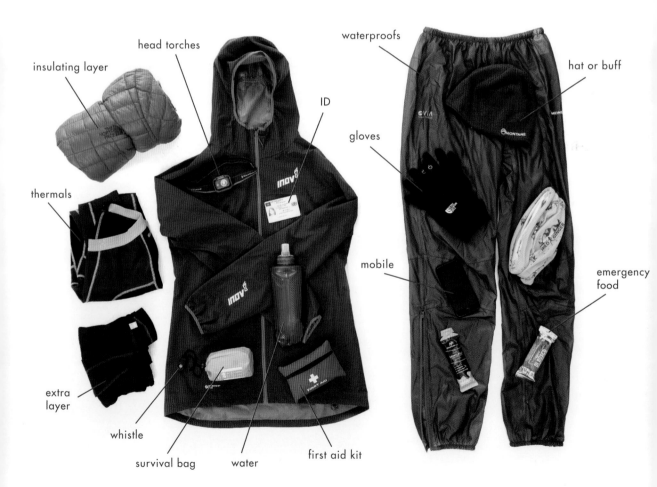

insulating layer

head torches

waterproofs

hat or buff

ID

gloves

thermals

mobile

emergency food

extra layer

whistle

survival bag

water

first aid kit

DON'T BE A DANGER

'There is the story of one runner turning up with "full body cover" ... for an Action Man rather than his own waterproof gear. The mandatory kit list is not a game of "What can I get away with?" It's vital you have your own packing list as well as the mandatory kit, with the right gear for your own safety if the weather turns bad or you have to stop. I can't recommend enough booking a mountain skills course if you are inexperienced.'

JAMES THURLOW, OPEN ADVENTURE RACE DIRECTOR

FULL-BODY WATERPROOF COVER

This means waterproof jacket and waterproof trousers, both with taped seams (see p. 143) and the jacket must have a hood (full-body). They may also specify how waterproof it must be with a Hydrostatic Head (HH) rating. This can usually be found online or contact the jacket manufacturer if it's an old product.

MOBILE PHONE

You might be carrying your smartphone anyway, but if you want to save weight, consider a tiny, old-school 40g (1^{1}/$_{2}$oz) phone that only does phoning and texting (remember those days?). Either way, make sure it is fully charged, or take a charger and portable battery if you plan to take a lot of photos, video or use the navigation, fitness tracking or music functions.

WATER

Races sometimes stipulate a minimum amount of water or water-carrying capacity to get you safely between aid stations, especially in hot climates or summer races. It's often 500ml–1 litre (17–34fl oz).

HEAD TORCHES

If there's a small chance you might finish in the dark, the RO may require everyone to carry a light head torch and they may specify the brightness – for example, 200 lumens minimum. If you are definitely running at night, they may ask you to carry either spare batteries or a spare head torch. A spare head torch is best – easier and quicker than faffing around changing batteries in the dark, but make sure it's at least 200 lumens or there's no point having it as you won't be able to see well enough to run unless the moon is full and the skies are super clear.

SURVIVAL BAG

There's a difference between a survival blanket that wraps around you like a cape, like at the London Marathon, and a survival bag that you can actually get one or two people inside, which is more like a very thin foil sleeping bag. Check which one is required and if there are any dimensions to consider.

WHISTLE

A lot of running packs have these on the chest strap clip or dangling from a shoulder strap, but if not, these are easily purchased from outdoor shops.

EMERGENCY FOOD

Some races require you to finish with a certain number of calories of emergency food, so a light but high-calorie energy bar is ideal for this.

FIRST AID KIT

The RO may specify what should go in a first aid kit (see opposite).

FULL-LENGTH LEGGINGS

Thermals to keep you warm should the weather turn polar.

EXTRA LAYER

This usually means a long-sleeved base layer made of technical, quick-drying material. The RO might specify a minimum weight to ensure it's warm enough.

INSULATING LAYER

A lightweight synthetic or down jacket for very cold situations. Always keep this in a dry bag so it doesn't get wet from your sweat or rain.

HAT, HEADBAND OR BUFF®

Pay close attention to what the RO allows here as there is often a great debate over whether a BUFF®-style tubular headband can also be called a hat, since although you can fold it into a lightweight hat, this is not considered enough by some ROs.

GLOVES

The RO might suggest lightweight or waterproof gloves, or a certain number of pairs. If you suffer with cold hands or Raynaud's syndrome (hands that get cold easily and are difficult to re-warm, becoming pale and numb), you may want to take warmer or more pairs of gloves than the mandatory kit list stipulates.

TRAIL HACK

SAVE A LIFE!

Defibrillators are available at many locations and come with easy instructions on use should someone collapse with a heart problem, so it's important to know where they are on your run. Use the Save a Life app to find out where the nearest AED (Automated, External Defibrillator) will be.

ID

It's a good idea to take your driving licence or photocopy of your passport ID page on a race, especially if you are racing abroad. Some races will state this, others may not. Check before you travel.

WHY NOT DO...

... a basic first aid course? They're fantastic for giving you the skills and confidence to cope with potentially life-threatening situations. Would you know how to save someone's life on the trail?

IT'S AN EMERGENCY!

In an emergency situation, call 999 and ask for Mountain Rescue. Keep calm, stay as warm as you can, give them all the details and follow their instructions. To indicate you need help, blow your whistle and/or flash your head torch six times, wait one minute, then repeat. This is the international distress signal. If waiting for a Search and Rescue helicopter, flash the light on the ground, not up at the pilots as this ruins their night vision. A rescue team will flash three times at you in response.

What's in a first aid kit?

A first aid kit isn't just for you – you never know when you might need to turn superhero and help someone on the trail. This is why it's a good idea to take a small one with you on every run if you're already carrying a pack as well as £10 cash just in case. A bit of extra weight is great training, after all. Using the first aid kit list from the mandatory kit section of race websites is a good place to start and here's what I have in mine for different levels of run.

BASIC FIRST AID KIT FOR LOW-LEVEL TRAILS CLOSE TO CIVILISATION

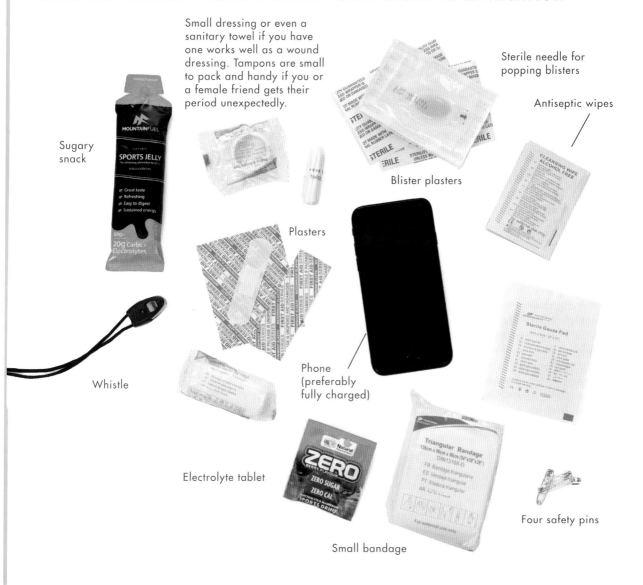

Small dressing or even a sanitary towel if you have one works well as a wound dressing. Tampons are small to pack and handy if you or a female friend gets their period unexpectedly.

Sterile needle for popping blisters

Antiseptic wipes

Blister plasters

Sugary snack

Plasters

Phone (preferably fully charged)

Whistle

Electrolyte tablet

Four safety pins

Small bandage

FULL FIRST AID KIT FOR REMOTE, HILLY OR MOUNTAINOUS TRAILS

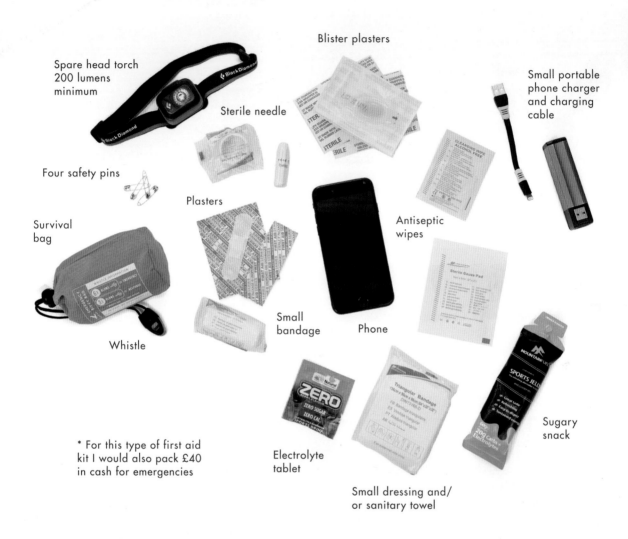

Spare head torch 200 lumens minimum

Blister plasters

Small portable phone charger and charging cable

Sterile needle

Four safety pins

Plasters

Antiseptic wipes

Survival bag

Small bandage

Phone

Whistle

* For this type of first aid kit I would also pack £40 in cash for emergencies

Electrolyte tablet

Sugary snack

Small dressing and/ or sanitary towel

- All of the items listed for low-level trails
- Survival bag (not blanket, you need to be able to get in it and preserve all the warmth rather than have it flapping around you)
- Small portable phone charger and charging cable

- More money if a taxi back might cost more than £10
- Spare head torch, 200 lumens minimum (I take another torch rather than spare batteries as it's fiddly, hard and slow to change them on the hill and you risk dropping and losing them)

NIGHT RUNNING KIT

Night running gives an exciting new angle on your usual trails, so grab a head torch and race for the hills to watch the sunset! If you're running on roads to get to your trails, it's also useful to don a bit of reflective gear, as described here.

HEAD TORCH
BRIGHTNESS
Lumens is the measure of brightness. Go for at least 200, but around 300–400 lumens is good for seeing enough of the trail at a fast pace for a few hours with not too heavy a battery. Be wary of torches promising huge 1000-lumen levels of brightness – it can be overkill. Super-bright lights will dazzle everyone around you, they don't work well in fog and the battery will either be heavier or it won't last as long. Beam pattern is more important for trail running.

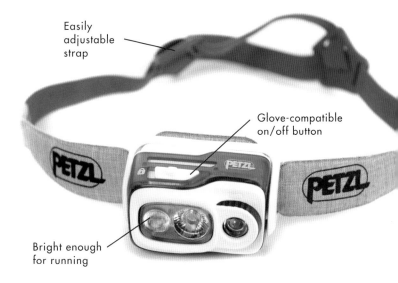

Easily adjustable strap

Glove-compatible on/off button

Bright enough for running

BEAM PATTERN
Look for a torch that enables you to switch between a bright, narrow spotlight beam to look into the distance and a wider flood beam so you can see the whole path using your peripheral vision without having to keep turning your head to keep lighting up different parts of the trail.

BATTERIES
Some torches take AAA and AA batteries, others take their own dedicated rechargeable lithium batteries and some take both, which is handy for long-distance or multi-day trail races. Lighter, less-bright torches store batteries behind the light on the forehead, while bigger, heavier batteries for a longer, brighter burn time tend to sit at the back of the head strap or in your pack via an extension wire.

BURN TIME
Check the technical specifications to see how long your torch burns for at certain levels of brightness. The brighter the light setting (the higher the lumens), the more battery power it eats, and vice versa.

TRAIL HACK

GET LIGHT RIGHT

A well-made head torch is an area not to scrimp on – when you're running on remote mountain trails you really need to be able to rely on it or you'll be stuck up there crawling on hands and knees to get down in the pitch-black (yes, this has happened to me). You can buy many cheap 1000-lumen imports but they actually do lie about the battery life and, more worryingly, I know of one case at Glenmore Lodge, Scottish National Outdoor Training Centre, where charging batteries have caught fire.

SETTINGS

Too many light settings can be confusing, so the best torches have a simple click-by-click succession of low, medium, high and flashing options, and possibly a boost button for a few seconds of super-bright light. You might also consider a red light option for night vision and a flashing red light for road safety. You may also/ alternatively want to use a red flashing light at the back for road safety, but make sure you can turn it off for night navigation races or else everyone will be able to follow you!

BUTTONS

Look for large buttons that can be used easily with gloves on, but not so easily pressed that they switch on in your bag. Travelling with the battery disconnected or the wrong way round is a good way to prevent this happening, but remember to reconnect before you start your run!

CUSTOMISATION

Some torches come with an app for customising the light settings. For some, this adds extra faff, but for others, it's a welcome upgrade. Check what settings you can only change via the app and make sure they're set correctly before you set off so you don't have to stop and get your phone out mid-run, especially on a wet, cold hillside.

REACTIVE LIGHTING

This is when the head torch brightness adjusts to the level it calculates that you need depending on the surrounding light. Some runners really like this for extending battery life while others find it can dim at unexpected times.

NIGHT RUNNING KIT

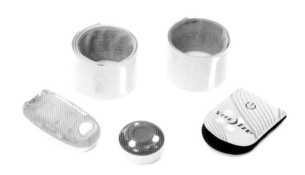

CLOTHING
Choose a light-coloured T-shirt or jacket in white or high-vis yellow, with plenty of reflective strips. The more reflective strips you have on your shorts and leggings the better too.

REFLECTIVE LED VEST
Look for a luminous yellow harness or mesh vest with reflective strips and flashing LED lights.

ARM AND ANKLE BANDS
Movement is what will get you detected so having luminous, reflective LED bands on your arms and ankles makes you highly visible.

SHOE LEDS
Clip-on LED lights for your shoes are a great idea as, like the above, the moving light will clearly show traffic where you are.

NIGHT RUNNING IS GREAT!

'I enjoy running in the dark. It adds a whole new layer of adventure to trail running. I love seeing a full moon or fireflies and running in cooler temperatures after a hot day. Navigation, foot placement and traffic safety are more difficult so I run on familiar paths on easier terrain. It can be scary when you hear forest sounds, spot eyes shining back in your head torch beam, or if you see an unexpected light, but mostly, trails are safer than roads. I do realise that as a large man I have less to worry about than my female counterparts, so if you are worried about night running, I would sign up to some night runs with a running club, go in a small group or run with a friend.'

JOHN GARDENER,
MARYLAND, USA

COLD-WEATHER RUNNING

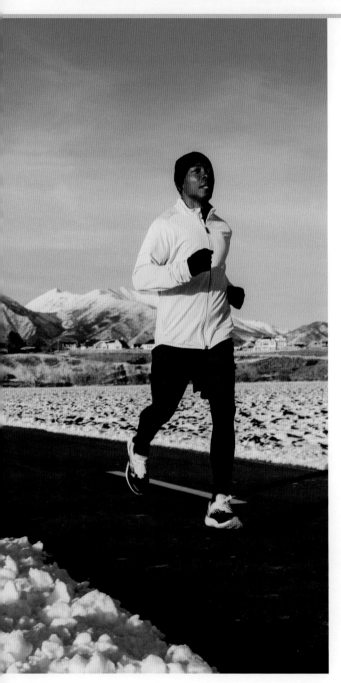

Cold out? Snowing even? Don't let the weather stop you from running. But do make sure you pack extra insulating gear and all the safety kit from p. 152. Put extra layers on before you get too cold, and if things get really gnarly, make the wise decision – stay at lower altitudes or turn back. Here's the kit you need in addition to or instead of your regular running kit to keep you enjoying your usual trails, however cold it gets.

THERMALS

Windproof, fleece-lined leggings and super-warm long-sleeved tops, layered over sweat-wicking vests or T-shirts, are the order of the day for runs in very cold weather or climates.

JACKET

It's always wise to run with a light jacket in case conditions change, but in winter you might want to wear a slightly heavier weight waterproof jacket to protect you from cold, wind, rain, sleet and snow.

INSULATING JACKET

Packing a super lightweight synthetic (man-made fibres) insulating jacket is prudent on very cold days in case you have to stop or slow down.

GLOVES

These range from slim to medium to full-on mountaineering gloves. I've been known to take all three types with me on one run – you never know how cold your hands might get and they are vital so you can pull all the zips and Velcro needed to keep the rest of you warm. Make them your priority!

HAT

Always take a light, fleecy, windproof hat to keep the chill off. Bobble-free makes it lighter and easier to pack.

BUFF®

A fantastically versatile tube of quick-wicking fabric that you can make into lots of different headwear, including a headband, neck warmer, balaclava and hat. I use this most often in headband mode to keep my ears warm.

WATERPROOF SOCKS

These are great in winter for keeping the feet warm while you thrash through freezing bogs and puddles. The higher up the ankle they go, the more protection they give.

RUNNING CRAMPONS OR ICE SPIKES

When tackling higher hill or mountain trails in icy conditions, you need these spikes over your trail shoes to dig into ice or hard-packed snow. The moment you feel out of your depth, however, do stay low level or turn back – respect snowy mountain trails and only run them if you are experienced.

ICE GRIPPERS

Great for icy pavements, these nifty over-shoe grippers will save you from slipping on low-level icy trails, such as canal towpaths, country parks and easy forest trails.

HAND WARMERS

If you know you get cold hands easily, particularly those with Raynaud's syndrome whose blood does not circulate effectively in cold weather, take a pair of hand warmers with you to pop in your gloves.

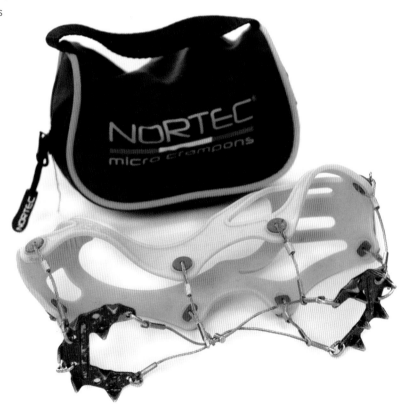

IS IT HYPOTHERMIA?

Being alert to the early signs of mild hypothermia is the best way to prevent it. These include:

- shivering
- cold, pale skin
- confusion
- tiredness
- slurred speech or mumbling
- fast breathing

Get the person warm and dry, try to persuade them to eat a sugary snack and sip a warm non-alcoholic drink if possible, put them into a survival bag if they're immobile, with another person for body heat if space allows, or add layers and keep moving to a place of warmth and safety (usually downhill). If a person stops shivering or passes out, urgent medical help is needed – call 999 and ask for Mountain Rescue.

Top tips for running in cold weather/climates

- Warm up for five minutes inside before venturing out.
- Keep your head and hands warm with gloves and a hat.
- Wear a technical, quick-wicking thermal base layer.
- Layer up your clothing so you can peel layers off as you warm up.
- Avoid stopping for too long and cooling down.
- Keep drinking – you breathe out moisture with every exhale.
- Start your run into the wind and finish with a tailwind.
- Make sure you're fully warmed before doing any speedwork.
- Get dry and warm quickly after running – this is where that big down jacket that you've stowed in the car comes in!

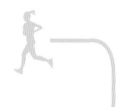

HOT-WEATHER RUNNING

It's tough to run in the heat, but the kit and tips here make it easier and safer. Stick to light-coloured clothing and add a few accessories.

LIGHTWEIGHT VEST AND SHORTS

Save your lightest-weight vest or T-shirt and shorts for hot weather. A T-shirt can be more comfy under a running pack than a vest, and helps more to prevent sunburn.

HEADBAND

You can get specially designed SPF 50 headbands (like a BUFF®) for sun protection. Dip them into a stream and wear them as a hat or headband to keep yourself cool.

CAP OR VISOR

A vital part of everyone's summer kit to help guard against sunstroke. Often, if it's not too sunny, you can get away without sunglasses under the peak of the cap.

SUNGLASSES

The best sunglasses wrap all the way around the eyes and don't slip off your nose when you get sweaty. Look for rubber grips at the nose and ears to prevent sliding. Cat 3 is a good level of lens protection, or photochromic, and I like to have a rosy tint to my lenses to make sunsets look even better. Watch out for polarised lenses as these make it very hard to read phone, watch and gadget screens.

SUNSCREEN

I use spray-on P20, which is a factor 15–50+ oil rather than a cream. You apply it once in the morning and it bonds with the skin to give sweat-resistant and waterproof UVA and UVB sun protection all day. Try not to get it on your clothes – it stains.

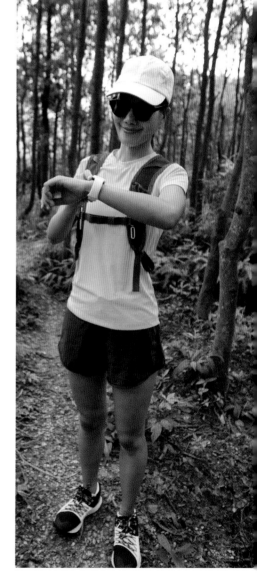

IS IT HEAT EXHAUSTION OR HEATSTROKE?

Heat exhaustion isn't usually serious if you can cool down within 30 minutes. Signs include:

- headache
- dizziness and confusion
- thirst
- loss of appetite
- nausea
- excessive sweating
- pale, clammy skin
- arm, leg and stomach cramps
- fast breathing or pulse
- a temperature of 38°C (100.4°F) or more

Move the person to a cool place, lie them down with feet raised, persuade them to drink plenty of water or electrolyte drink, cool their skin with water and fan them. Call 999 and ask for Mountain Rescue if they move into heatstroke – if they are no better after 30 minutes, feel hot and dry, are not sweating, have a temperature of more than 40°C (104°F), have rapid breath or shortness of breath, are still confused, have a fit, lose consciousness or become unresponsive.

TRAIL HACK

GET CHEAP SUNNIES

I'm always losing or breaking my sunnies so if that's you, go for a £30 pair – they're perfectly adequate and cause much less heartache!

Top tips for running in hot weather/climates

- Have a cool shower and wet your hair before you run.
- Avoid running at the hottest times of the day.
- Run slower – don't expect to be able to run as fast.
- Drink regular sips of water mixed with electrolytes (salts).
- Wear breathable clothing – light-coloured, loose fabrics.
- Wear a cap and sunglasses to create your own shade.
- Dip your cap into streams or water at aid stations as you pass.
- Spray yourself with water or crocodile roll in streams.
- Wrap a BUFF® round your wrist and keep wetting it.
- Familiarise yourself with the first signs of heat exhaustion, and stop and get into the shade if you experience them.

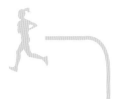

RUNNING POLES

Running poles can help ease the strain on your legs and knee joints, especially on longer trail races with smooth, wide paths. They're also great for balance, so if you're expecting a lot of river crossings, definitely pack those poles. Look for carbon options weighing 130–200g (5–8oz) each, and check what length they fold down to as that will determine how easy they are to carry.

ARE THEY ALLOWED?
Before you take your poles to a race check the rules; not all events allow competitors to use poles, especially fell (mountain) races in the north of England and Scotland.

ADJUST THE GRIP
Slide your hand through the pole strap from underneath and grip the pole handle. Adjust the Velcro or slider on the strap so it supports your hand comfortably.

GET THE RIGHT LENGTH
Now stand on flattish ground with your pole next to your shoe. You're aiming for a 90-degree bend at the elbow, so adjust the height of the pole or measure accordingly if you're looking at fixed-length poles. With adjustable poles, look for a quick-release clip rather than the ones you have to unscrew as these are really hard to use, especially with cold hands.

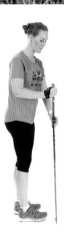

HOW TO RUN WITH POLES

1. Be aware of people around you and keep 1–2m (3.3–6.6ft) away so as not to stab others in the heels or poke them in the head as you lift your arms to climb a stile.

2. Swing the poles alternately as you run, planting each one just ahead of your leading foot and push off when it is behind you, helping to propel you forwards. You can also use both poles at a time to long jump smoothly over rocks and puddles (this is great fun to do!).

3. Scan the path ahead for pole placements to avoid catching the pole tips between rocks, wooden slats and boggy bits.

CROSS RIVERS SAFELY

Use your running poles to help you balance during river crossings, but never underestimate the power of flowing water. Always go upstream to a bridge or shallower crossing place if you can. Never cross deep, wide, fast-flowing rivers unless you and your group are very experienced.

YOUR OPINIONS – RUNNING POLES OR CHEAT STICKS?

'I used them on the 50-mile [80km] UTS [Ultra-Trail Snowdonia] this year – found them VERY useful! I used them on the long, steep uphills to give a bit of extra stability and help when (very) tired. I used them on some of the flatter sections to help keep a rhythm. They were sometimes useful when descending too.'

Gordon Saxby, Surrey

'Terrain needs to be Goldilocks [ideal condition] for cheat sticks. Too muddy and they get stuck. Too rocky or gnarly and they're uselessly slipping about. If up and down on well maintained paths then they're OK, but who wants to run only on well-maintained paths...?'

Tommy Hughes, Norfolk

'I have hypermobility and poles are a life-saver as they take strain off my joints, which are already working twice as hard to stay in position. I really hate it when people call them cheat sticks.'

Jodie Haggerty, near Chester

'Never used them as I only really do events in Scotland where until very recently they were banned. I might get around to trying them one day but if doing very technical hills, they wouldn't be useful.'

Craig Beattie, Dundee

ANTI-CHAFE CREAM

For longer distances, you might find various parts of you begin to rub uncomfortably against each other, so a tube of sports lube and/or nipple tape for runners could be a gift from heaven.

DRY BAGS

Keeping spare kit dry in winter is essential, so pop it into airtight, sealable sandwich bags or invest in some more robust dry bags from an outdoor shop.

HEADPHONES

If you want to listen to music or podcasts (great motivation for longer runs), it's worth investing in some water-resistant, wireless headphones.

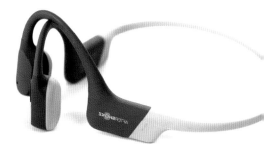

ARMBAND FOR SMARTPHONE

These are great for carrying your phone on shorter runs when you don't need a pack. You can usually fit a credit card and key in them too.

COMPASS

If you want to start planning your own trail routes in the hills and mountains, and are doing navigation events, a compass will help you find your way, especially in misty weather.

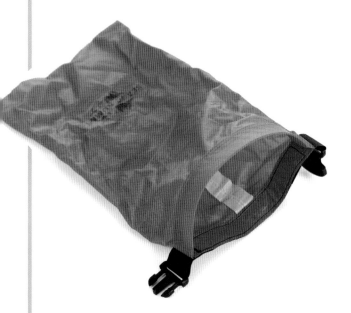

TRAIL HACK

KEEP HANDS WARM

In cold weather, keep your gloves on to adjust metal poles as they can supercool your hands really quickly.

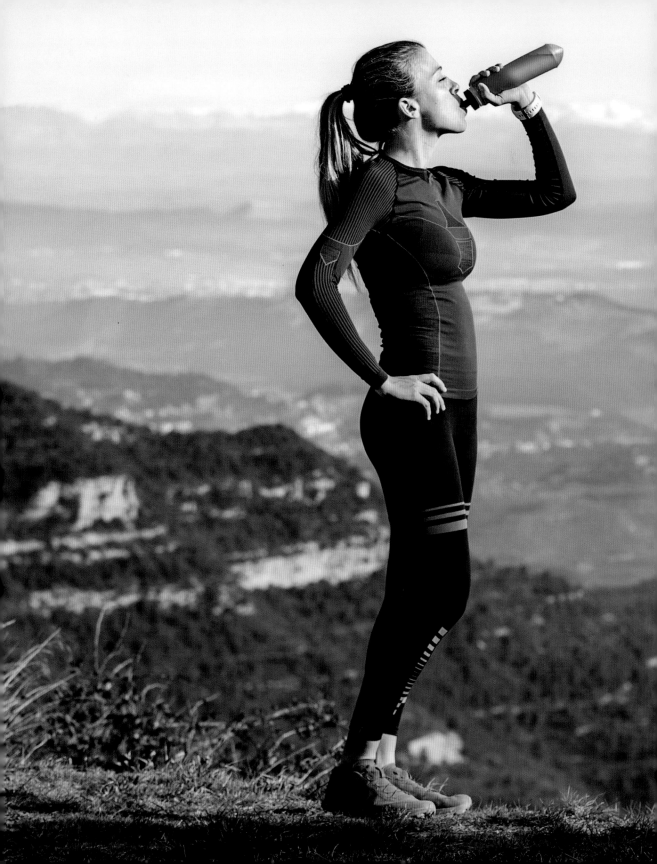

6

NUTRITION AND HYDRATION

Cake and beer are a very good reason to run, but having
a healthy, nutritious diet works wonders for your
performance without having to do any extra training.
Here's what to eat when, why, and the most delicious recipes.

BASIC FUELLING

Food and drink are the whole reason we run, hey? To add treats to our usual healthy, nutritious diet of fruit and veg… Here are some delicious, healthy recipes for breakfast, lunch and dinner that will keep your energy levels high for your best performance. There are also portable snacks to keep you running strong and foods to speed up your recovery.

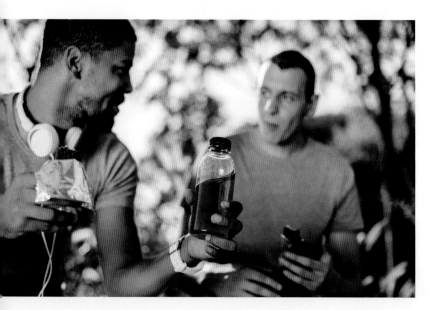

HEALTHIER FUEL = BETTER RUNNING

Fuelling up with healthy, nutritious food and drink should be everyone's goal wherever you're at on your running journey. For the healthiest weight and best running performance you want to eat a highly nutritious diet filled with many different-coloured vegetables and fruit; protein from lean meat, fish, legumes, pulses and tofu; some carbohydrates (quick- or slow-release depending on the situation). Cut back on processed high-fat and high-sugar foods. The great news is that runners can afford to eat more than sedentary people and during or after long trail runs you will benefit from eating those high-fat, high-sugar foods a healthy diet wouldn't usually contain (such as cake, biscuits, sugary drinks, pies and pastries). However, these should still be a treat reserved for after really intense or long runs and races.

HEALTHY EVERYDAY FUEL

All of these lush, healthy things should be on your plate regularly, filling you with high-quality nutrition with plenty of energy, vitamins and minerals. Eating and drinking these foods will make your body as healthy as it can be for best running performance, illness resistance and recovery.

PROTEIN

Protein from meat, fish, pulses, dairy products and nuts helps muscles repair and adapt to training.

FAT
Fat is crucial for energy, cell membrane function, hormonal control and absorbing vitamins A, D, E and K. The healthiest versions are unsaturated, found in avocados, olive oil, nuts, seeds and oily fish.

CARBOHYDRATES (CARBS)
Carbs such as potatoes, chickpeas, rice, oats and bananas are the body's main fuel source, particularly for high-intensity exercise and anything else that requires energy, such as brain function.

VITAMINS
Vitamins are organic substances found in all natural foods and all 13 play a vital role in making sure your body functions well, from bone health to healing, converting food into energy and boosting your immune system.

MINERALS
Minerals are inorganic substances formed naturally in the earth and include iron, calcium, potassium, sodium, magnesium and zinc. They are essential to many different body processes, such as oxygen transport, muscle contraction, bone health and nerve transmission.

LONG RUN OR RACE FUEL
Rather than calling this pile of goodies 'unhealthy' food, us runners recognise that high-fat and/or high-sugar foods have their uses in powering us on our long runs and races. However, if you're eating or drinking a lot of these items on non-running days, swap them for more of the healthy fuel.

TRAIL HACK

DITCH THE GUILT

Don't ban yourself from eating tempting, high-fat and/or high-sugar foods such as chocolate, biscuits, pies, cakes and sweets. Focus instead on feeding your body highly nutritious fuel and you'll feel full from nutrient-rich sources and naturally have fewer cravings for unhealthy foods.

MEET THE EXPERT
A selection of the recipes in this section come from sports nutritionist Anita Bean, author of *The Runner's Cookbook*. Anita's book contains more than 100 delicious recipes to fuel your running as well as advice on optimising recovery and hydration, whether high-fat/low-carb diets really work, how to achieve your ideal racing weight, fuel for races and more. Anita says: 'I've been working with athletes from Olympic level to club runners for more than 25 years and what you eat has a massive impact on your health and running performance. A good diet gives you the energy and nutrients you need to train harder, perform better, recover quicker and stay free of injury and illness. All the quick, easy and tasty recipes in my book will help you do this.'
www.anitabean.co.uk

FOOD MYTHS BUSTED

Especially on social media, you can see a lot of hype about the latest superfood and slimming diet, performance-enhancing potions and muscle-building must-eats. In the main, it's best to take each of these with a large pinch of salt and stick to a healthy, high-quality, balanced diet rich in nutrients. Here, some of the main areas about diet that cause confusion are explained by qualified and registered sports nutritionist Anita Bean, author of *The Runner's Cookbook*.

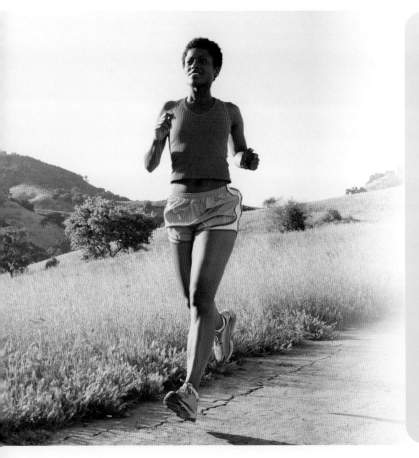

MYTH:
Sugar is bad for runners

BUSTED:
Sugar is a great source of quick energy before, during and after long runs and intense workouts, so on these occasions it's actually a very useful and good thing for runners. However, part of the myth is true: it's bad for your teeth, and eating too much of it can lead to weight gain, insulin resistance and type 2 diabetes. As long as you use small amounts (30–60g/1¼–2½ oz per hour) as a fuel source just for exercise, it's not bad for you.

MYTH:
I need to go low carb!

BUSTED:
There is a lot of confusing information in the running world about Low Carb High Fat (LCHF or HFLC) diets. This diet dramatically reduces your carbohydrate intake so your body is forced to burn spare fat for fuel instead, known as ketosis or keto. While this can be useful for initial weight loss for those who need it, low-carb diets can be both hard and detrimental for runners to maintain due to their increased energy requirements and the need for carbs in the recovery process.

There has also been a trend for longer-distance (ultra) runners to take this approach to train their bodies to use fat reserves as fuel so they don't need to carry as much to eat. With gradual practice, a lower-carb intake can work for slow running, but there is no scientific evidence that it works for running fast, so you can lose speed over shorter distances. It can also depress your immune system and reduce recovery rates, and once you have no fat reserves left, ketosis leads to muscle breakdown as your body searches for fuel from its last resort: protein.

Having interviewed many, many top athletes from all over the world about their nutrition, I've discovered that most don't overthink food or stick rigidly to any special diets. They mostly eat a normal healthy diet (see chapter 6), perhaps plant-based (see vegan myths opposite), and have a couple of gels or snacks on long (two hours or more) runs or races.

MYTH:
Being vegan is best for runners

BUSTED:
Over the last decade, many top athletes have turned to a vegan (no animal products, i.e. meat or dairy) or plant-based (mainly plants, but not fully vegan) diet. It is a good way to reduce your footprint on the planet and respect animal welfare, but vegans have to make sure they eat enough vitamin B12, calcium, vitamin D and iron – all of which are found easily in eggs, oily fish, dairy products and meat. Multivitamins, supplements, algae and seaweed products help with this.

MYTH:
Vegan runners don't get enough protein

BUSTED:
This is a total myth as it's very easy for runners to get plenty of protein from beans, lentils, tofu, grains, nuts and seeds. However, there is a legitimate concern that plant protein is less easily absorbed and used by the body, so vegans need to eat a wide variety of meat- and dairy-free foods containing protein so they get the full range of essential amino acids.

MYTH:
I need to eat loads of pasta before a race

BUSTED:
Carb loading came into fashion with pre-marathon pasta parties a few decades ago, but although you need your muscles to be well stocked with glycogen before a big race, this is very easy to do with a carb-rich meal of any kind the night before. Provided that you're not totally starving and have tapered (not exercised much) the week before an event, a large, satisfying portion should be enough to top up those muscles nicely.

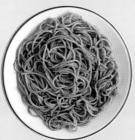

MYTH:
I'll get cramp if I don't eat enough salt

BUSTED:
People have popped salt tablets for years in the hope of staving off cramp – where the muscle (usually the calf for runners) contracts involuntarily and won't relax. However, surprisingly, there isn't much evidence that cramp is caused by dehydration and lack of electrolytes (mineral salts, such as sodium, chloride, potassium and magnesium). Cramp is likely to occur in tired muscles or where there is a muscle imbalance, so fuel up properly before running, avoid setting off too fast and work on your overall strength and technique.

MYTH:
Losing weight will make me run faster

BUSTED:
Yes, carrying less weight does allow you to speed up, but not if you lose more than 500g (1lb 1oz) per week as this may lead to too much energy and muscle loss. Thinness does not always equal strength or fitness; I've beaten many a slimmer runner from parkrun to trail marathon, and even beaten my own times after putting on half a stone. If you are not dangerously overweight (talk to your GP for guidelines), forget obsessing about weight. Make your goal long-term healthy fuel without overeating most of the time, because the more severe your weight-loss diet, the less sustainable it will be. With a truly healthy diet, fat loss will happen slowly and so will your increase in speed. There are no quick fixes or shortcuts to a long-term healthy, sustainable diet with sensible, sustainable training.

MYTH:

I need to run on an empty stomach to lose weight

BUSTED:

Actually, your total energy balance over days, weeks and months matters the most when it comes to weight loss, not whether or not you run on empty. If you run faster – for example, before breakfast when you haven't eaten for perhaps 10–12 hours – you will be forcing your body to burn fat. However, because burning fat for fuel takes longer for your body to do, you'll have less glycogen in your muscles and you will only be able to run slowly, so you may actually burn fewer calories per minute due to a less intense run. It's a bit of a mind game, so it's simpler to understand the following: if your total energy (measured in calories) coming in is less than the energy you are expending (by simply being alive and also exercising), you will use up fat stores and therefore hopefully lose weight. But also, do bear in mind that muscle is denser than fat, and therefore weighs more, so becoming a healthier, better runner isn't necessarily all about weight loss.

MYTH:

I'll get the trots if I run fast!

BUSTED:

This is a terrible affliction: suddenly finding yourself in urgent need of a poo while running even though you didn't feel like one before you set off. You feel it more if you are trying to run fast, such as when at parkrun or doing speedy efforts up a hill, because your gut is being shaken around, blood flow is being redirected to your muscles, you might be becoming dehydrated, and your stress hormones are gearing you up for fight or flight. Symptoms include gut pain, bloating, nausea, heartburn, farting, burping and, in the worst cases, vomiting and diarrhoea. Take a note of any foods that trigger this, do a warm-up with some 20–30-second faster efforts then pop to the loo, cut back on high-fibre foods the day before, stay hydrated, don't eat too much sugar and practise eating and drinking on longer runs.

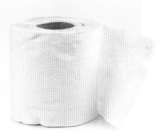

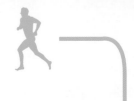

FUEL TIMELINE

What to eat when is particularly important when you're racing. This timeline is a good guideline to keep you full of energy and well hydrated during running, and to speed up your recovery and ward off illness and injury afterwards.

DAY BEFORE
Eat normally and make sure you are well hydrated using the info on pp. 190–192.

NIGHT BEFORE
Eat a healthy meal rich in carbs, protein and good-quality nutrients, such as fish, chicken, tofu and chickpeas with rice and vegetables. There's no need to stuff yourself – being fully satisfied will ensure all your energy stores are completely topped up. It's best not to try anything you haven't eaten before in case it disagrees with you, so if you're in a different country maybe tonight is not the night to try the thing you don't quite understand on the menu...

TWO HOURS BEFORE
It's best to eat two hours before your start time so your body has time for digestion. This is often breakfast time, so have some porridge with honey or a couple of slices of toast with eggs – whatever you are used to eating before running is a good idea here. If

it's not breakfast, have a small, plain meal, such as an omelette, chicken sandwich or some vegetable rice. For more ideas, see pp. 178–179.

THIRTY MINUTES BEFORE
Especially if it's a long race over 90 minutes long, you might want to have a small snack on the start line, such as an energy bar, flapjack or gel, as a final top-up for your muscles' glycogen reserves.

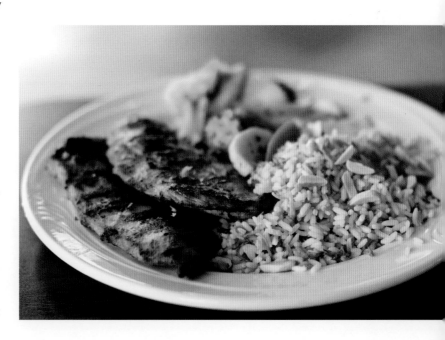

DURING

During short, flat-out races such as a 5k or 10k you may not have time or need to eat or drink anything as your muscles hold enough fuel for 60–90 minutes of running. However, once you reach the 90-minute mark and longer you will benefit from a small carb-rich (sugary) snack every 20–40 minutes. It is recommended that you consume 30–60g (1$^1/_4$–2$^1/_2$ oz) carbs per hour, which is 6–12 Jelly Babies. Drink to thirst with water, electrolyte, isotonic or energy drinks as per pp. 191–192.

WITHIN TWO HOURS AFTER

After your race, first make sure you rehydrate by steadily sipping at a pint of water, squash or electrolyte drink (see p. 191). If you aren't eating a meal within this time, speed up your recovery with a snack containing 3:1 carbs and protein (see pp. 184–185 for ideas).

THAT EVENING

Depending on when your race finishes, you might have missed lunch and be straight on to dinner. Have whatever you fancy! Have a beer! It's good to keep it healthy (see pp. 182–183 for ideas) but if you've been craving fish and chips for months, reward yourself now; life is for living!

THE NEXT DAY

Ease back into your regular healthy eating, making sure you eat plenty of protein (such as lean meat, fish, tofu, pulses and quinoa) combined with carbs for recovery.

TRAIL HACK

NO BONKING!

Avoid bonking or 'hitting the wall' on race day by remembering to eat a small carb snack like Jelly Babies after 90 minutes of running has passed. Hitting the wall is when you completely run out of energy, usually at around miles 18–20 (kilometres 29–32) on a marathon or after about three–four hours of running.

MY STORY

DON'T COPY ME!

'My cousin and I do races all over the world together and always have a slap-up meal from a local restaurant the night beforehand, tasting all the dishes we've never heard of before. In the past we've tried snails dripping in oil in Barcelona, sausages the size of your arm in Slovenia and the world's hottest curry in New York. So far, I've never suffered from our pre-race feasting, but I would never advise anyone else to do the same for obvious reasons!'

VASSOS ALEXANDER,
VIRGIN RADIO SPORTS PRESENTER

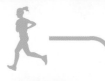

BREAKFASTS WORTH WAKING UP FOR

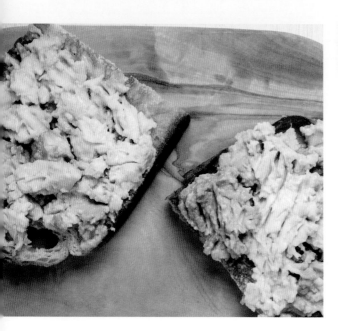

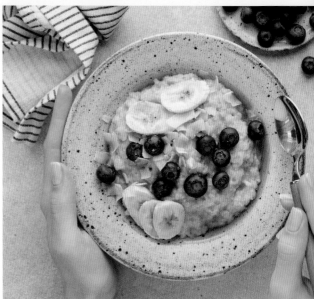

SMASHED AVOCADO JOY
Very hipster, and healthy too.

MAKE IT
Toast 2 slices of sourdough bread, spread with 1 mashed avocado, add a pinch of salt and a squirt of lemon juice to taste. Chomp!

VARY IT
Make proper guacamole first, with garlic, chilli, chopped tomatoes, salt and pepper and a squeeze of lemon juice. Or cheat – buy a tub of guacamole and spread it on!

CLAIRE'S POWER PORRIDGE
A great mix of carbs and protein to keep you full all morning.

MAKE IT
Mix 50g (2oz) porridge oats with 1 sliced banana, 1 handful of raisins, 1 tbsp seeds, 1 tbsp desiccated coconut, 1 tsp peanut butter, 1 tsp honey and about 125ml (4^1/4 fl oz) milk, then microwave for 2–3 minutes, stirring halfway through the cooking time.

VARY IT
Add different fruits, such as pear, blackberries or blueberries for seasonal variety. Freezer fruits work well too – just microwave first to thaw before adding to the cooked porridge.

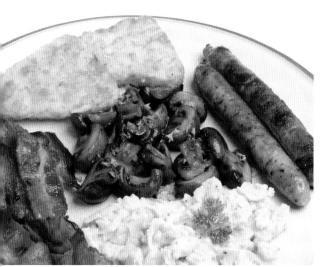

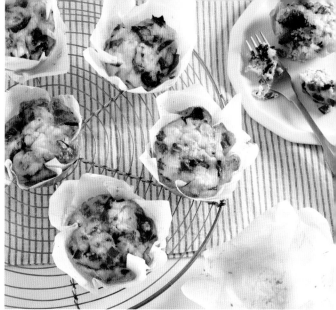

HEALTHY BRUNCH

A wonderful stomach-filler mid-morning after a long run or race.

MAKE IT

Get 2 sausages and/or bacon going under the grill, chop 200g (8oz) mushrooms, and whisk 2 eggs. Fry the mushrooms in butter until brown. Scoop onto a plate and leave under the grill to keep warm. When the sausages/bacon look done, scramble the eggs in the mushroom pan (give it a wipe if you're fussy) for a couple of minutes. Plate everything up and indulge.

VARY IT

I'm a big fan of veggie sausages for this. Add ½ grilled tomato and potato cakes or hash browns. Mop your plate with toast, or have jam on toast afterwards and call it pudding.

ANITA BEAN'S BREAKFAST EGG MUFFINS

Great for when you're on the go. *The Runner's Cookbook* author Anita Bean says: 'These healthy muffins are basically mini frittatas, packed full of protein and also a great way of getting in some veg.'

MAKE IT

Preheat the oven to 180°C/160°C fan/gas mark 4, grease a 12-hole muffin tin. Mix 6 eggs in a bowl and stir in ¼ onion, 6 cherry tomatoes, ½ handful of spinach, ½ seeded red pepper, 40g (1½ oz) crumbled feta and a pinch of salt and pepper. Divide the mixture between the holes of the muffin tin and bake for 15–20 minutes until golden and set. Tip the muffins onto a wire rack to cool, then eat! They'll keep refrigerated in an airtight container for three days.

VARY IT

Use different veg like mushrooms, yellow pepper and courgettes.

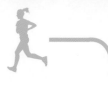

QUICK-AND-EASY LUNCHES

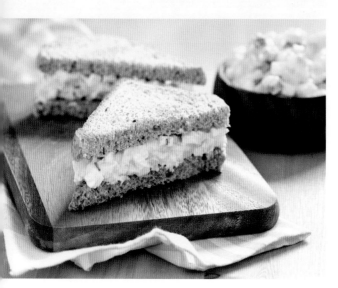

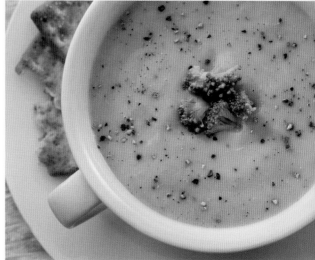

JOSS NAYLOR'S LUSCIOUS SANDWICH

According to legendary fell runner Joss Naylor, a moist sandwich is best for long runs of more than four hours. 'You need a sandwich that's luscious, good to get down and easy to digest,' says Joss. Here's his favourite...

MAKE IT

Hard-boil a couple of eggs, cool, peel, mix with 1 tbsp mayo and a pinch of salt. Use as a sandwich filling between slices of crusty brown bread.

VARY IT

Add your own favourite luscious sandwich boosters, such as chopped chives, cream cheese, mango chutney, houmous, guacamole, salsa, nacho cheese dip, or a daring combination of three.

BROCCOLI AND STILTON SOUP

Surely the best winter warmer and one of the most simple batch foods to cook at the weekend and bag up in the freezer. Double these quantities to make a bigger batch.

MAKE IT

Fry up 1 large chopped onion in a dash of oil until soft, then add 1 diced large potato. Fry for five minutes, then throw in 2 chopped broccolli heads, cover with boiling water and add 2 veg stock cubes. Cook for 15–20 minutes or until the veg is soft. Blend it up, then crumble in 300g (10^{1}/2 oz) Stilton. Divide into plastic containers and freeze.

VARY IT

Try adding a leek, a small head of cauliflower and some celery sticks instead of one of the broccoli heads.

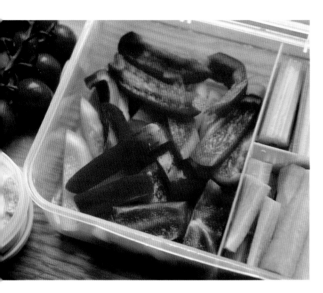

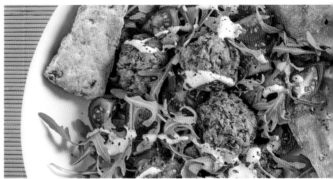

EASIEST-EVER SALAD

Who knows what cutlery there'll be at work?
Make healthy crudités, ready to dip and eat.

MAKE IT

Chop 1 medium carrot, 1–2 celery and carrot
sticks and $1/2$ seeded pepper into batons and line
them up in your plastic container. Add some
baby gem lettuce leaves, baby sweetcorn, sugar
snaps and cherry tomatoes. Take a small tub of
houmous to dip them in.

VARY IT

Take different dips, such as salsa, guacamole,
sour cream and nacho cheese.

ANITA BEAN'S BAKED FALAFELS

The Runner's Cookbook author Anita Bean says: 'These
are healthier than the traditional recipes as the falafels
are baked rather than fried. Chickpeas are a fantastic
source of fibre, protein, zinc, iron and probiotics that
feed the beneficial bacteria in your gut.'

MAKE IT

Preheat the oven to 200°C/180°C fan/gas mark 6
and lightly oil a baking tray. Blend up a 400g (14oz)
can of drained chickpeas with $1/2$ chopped onion,
2 crushed garlic cloves, 2 tsp ground coriander, 1
tsp ground cumin, a handful of fresh coriander, $1/2$
tsp baking powder, 1 tbsp plain flour, 2 tbsp water,
the zest of $1/2$ lemon and 1 tbsp olive oil, aiming
for a stiff paste. Spoon 16 balls of mixture onto
the baking tray, brush with oil and bake for 18–20
minutes, until golden. Serve with tahini yoghurt,
rocket, baby tomatoes and a warmed pitta bread.

VARY IT

I've used butter beans instead of chickpeas or half/
half, and experimented by adding sweetcorn and
peppers to the falafel mixture for more moisture.

NUTRITIOUS 20-MINUTE DINNERS

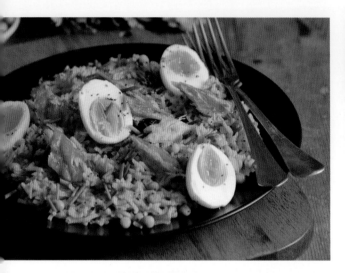

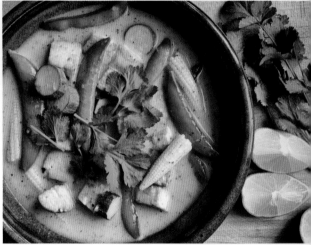

ALMOST KEDGEREE

This is a super-quick, easy meal for two when you haven't got any fresh ingredients and you're fighting the urge to order takeaway.

MAKE IT

Pop 2 pieces of frozen smoked haddock in the microwave for 3 minutes, or steam it in a pan. Microwave 300g (10½ oz) peas for 3 minutes, then microwave a packet of microwave pilau rice for 2 minutes. Mix it all together on two plates and scoff!

VARY IT

Of course, a real kedgeree contains hard-boiled eggs, fresh chives and lemon juice, so do add these if you have the ingredients to hand.

THAI GREEN CURRY

Great for batch cooking in a ginormous pan.

MAKE IT

Put enough rice or noodles on for tonight's meal. Chop up as much colourful, crunchy veg as you think you can get in your biggest pan – e.g. carrots, peppers, baby sweetcorn, French beans, sugar snaps, courgette slices, mangetouts and broccoli florets. Fry 1 chopped large onion and crushed garlic to taste, add 1–2 tbsp proper Thai green curry paste, stir, then add the harder veg first, followed by the softer veg, and stir to combine. When the veg looks almost cooked, add 1–2 x 400g (14oz) tins coconut milk depending on how big a batch cook you're doing and how much sauce you prefer. Simmer for 5–10 minutes but try not to let the veg go too soft. Serve with rice or noodles.

VARY IT

Try a Thai red curry sauce next time.

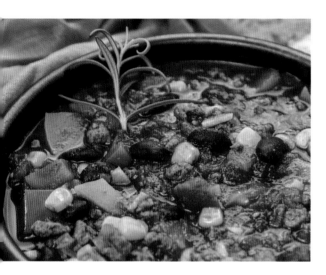

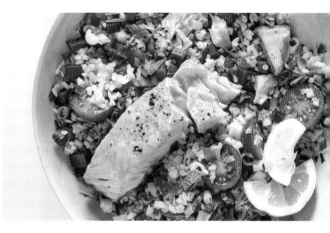

COWBOY HASH

I learned to make this in home economics at school with beef mince and have been batch cooking this cheap and cheerful chilli in various guises ever since. It tastes even better on day two.

MAKE IT
Fry 1 large chopped onion and crushed garlic cloves to taste in a dash of oil until soft. Add 1kg (2lb 3oz) Quorn or beef mince and fry until golden. Add $1/2$ bottle red wine and simmer. Add 2 chopped peppers, 1 tin each of sweetcorn, kidney beans and baked beans, 3 x 400g (14oz) tins of chopped tomatoes, 1 small tin tomato purée, 2 veg stock cubes and a pinch of dried mixed herbs. Simmer for 5–10 minutes, or longer if you have time. Serve with anything – rice, spaghetti or a baked potato.

VARY IT
Vary the beans and add more of them.

ANITA BEAN'S SALMON TABBOULEH

This is a fresh and delicious addition to your repertoire, especially for summer evenings and contains a more unusual grain. *The Runner's Cookbook* author Anita Bean says: 'This Lebanese salad is a great source of fibre, iron, zinc, vitamin C, protein and essential omega-3 fats, fantastic for recovery after running.'

MAKE IT
Cook 2 portions of bulgur wheat according to the packet instructions, then drain. Meanwhile, chop 2 spring onions, $1/2$ seeded pepper, small handfuls of mint and parsley, and 100g (4oz) cherry tomatoes. Squeeze the juice of $1/2$ lemon over 2 pieces of salmon, fry in a very hot pan for two minutes, then turn and fry the skin side for 2–3 minutes or until just cooked through. Add the veg and herbs to the cooked and drained bulgur wheat, then serve with the salmon on top and a slice of lemon to squeeze over.

VARY IT
Try with couscous or quinoa too.

HEALTHY SNACK IDEAS

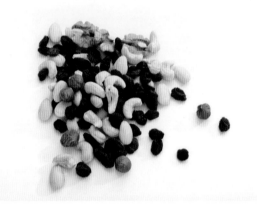

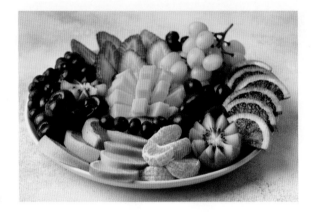

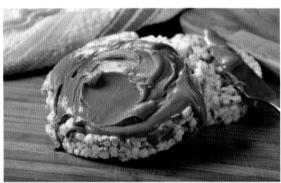

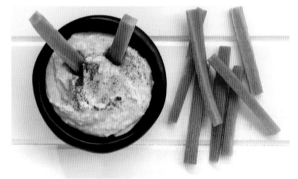

1 NUTS AND RAISINS

Great for energy, nutrients and good fats, a handful of nuts is a useful, easy snack at any time.

2 RICE CAKES WITH PEANUT BUTTER

You can also use corncakes and/or Marmite. Make a sandwich with them if you need them to be portable.

3 FRESH FRUIT

Fruit is my test for whether I'm actually hungry between meals or just a bit bored! If you fancy sugary chocolate, biscuits and sweets but not a sumptuous slice of mango, a handful of blueberries, an apple or a banana, you can't be that hungry, so have a cup of tea instead.

4 CRUDITÉS

Absolutely delicious and more filling than you think, crunchy carrots dipped in houmous are especially good for combatting crisp cravings. Cucumbers, sugar snaps or peppers dipped in guacamole or cottage cheese are also a good choice.

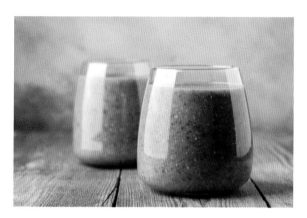

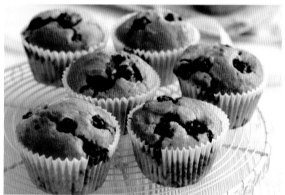

5 DISGUISED VEG SMOOTHIE

Healthy veg is even easier to consume if you drink it whizzed up with sweet fruit.

MAKE IT

Whizz up 1 cored, chopped apple, a few chunks of frozen mango, 1 chopped carrot, 2 handfuls of spinach, 3 broccoli florets and a hunk of fresh root ginger (to taste). Add water, soy, nut or normal milk until it's the desired consistency. Add more apple or apple juice and less veg if it's not sweet enough for you.

VARY IT

Experiment with different veg, adding smaller amounts of really strong flavoured ones – for example, beetroot, and sweetening them up with other fruits such as berries.

6 ANITA BEAN'S BLUEBERRY MUFFINS

Hallelujah! A healthier muffin snack for runners! *The Runner's Cookbook* author Anita Bean says, "These muffins are a far cry from the coffee shop version, which are loaded with fat and sugar."

MAKE IT

Preheat the oven to 200°C/180°C fan/gas mark 6 and line a muffin tin with 12 paper cases. Mix 75g (3oz) brown sugar or honey, 75g (3oz) olive oil spread, 2 eggs, 1 tsp vanilla extract, 4 tbsp milk and 100ml (3.4fl oz) plain low-fat Greek yoghurt in a bowl. Sift in 200g (8oz) self-raising flour and mix. Fold in 125g (5oz) fresh blueberries or 75g (3oz) dried blueberries. Divide the mixture into the cases, then bake for 20 minutes until risen and golden.

VARY IT

Try with dried or seasonal fruits like raisins, apricots, raspberries and blackberries.

LONG-DISTANCE RACE FUEL

If you're eating sensibly most days, you won't usually need to eat any food on runs of 90 minutes or less. However, whatever the length of your run, you might wish to have a small snack in your pocket for sudden dips in energy or unexpected navigational excitement... For runs planned to last more than two hours, definitely pack a snack, using a mix of sweet and savoury foods.

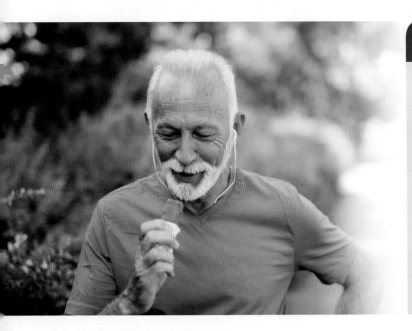

TRAIL HACK

ECO SNACKS

Instead of using new ziplock bags for your trail snacks, you can be more eco-friendly (and save pennies) by using the plastic packaging from other items, such as cherry tomatoes, dried fruits and nuts, crisps, wraps and even magazines or junk mail.

FIND NEW FOOD IDEAS

To find new long-distance food ideas, I walk down the supermarket aisles I never usually go down – such as the sweets, chocolate, biscuit, crisps and cake aisles – lest I be tempted into buying unhealthy food. Look for things that won't go off quickly in hot weather, be inedible if squashed or broken, that can be made into bite-sized pieces and that are digested easily.

HOW TO FUEL UP ON THE MOVE

Practise eating and drinking during your run. Pack snacks in an easily accessible pocket in your clothing or running pack and carry your liquids in soft bottles up front or in a hydration bladder. After 60–90 minutes, take small bites and sips every 20–40 minutes to top up your energy supplies regularly. If you wait until you are very hungry or extremely thirsty to eat and drink, it can be too late and adversely affect your mood and performance.

JELLY BABIES

The original source of running fuel. Chewy, sugary, fruit-flavoured sweets like this are a fantastic bite-sized pick-me-up mid-race and don't mind being squashed or getting sweaty in your pocket.

DRIED FRUIT

Nature's sweets are an easy, nutritious option. Particularly run-friendly are succulent ready-to-eat apricots and Medjool dates – they're delicious, light (especially if you pre-stone the dates) and slide down easily in a couple of bites.

JAM AND PEANUT BUTTER SARNIES

Make these with the ratio of jam to peanut butter you most enjoy, on white bread for quicker digestion and energy absorption, then cut into quarters for bite-sized snacking mid-run.

HOT CROSS BUNS

You can eat these plain and they come in all types of flavours now, such as chocolate orange, but if it's not too warm outside, my fave is a buttered original bun. Cut it in four and enjoy snacking on this soft, raisin-y delight. Malt loaf also should be mentioned here, treated similarly.

DARREN JOYNES' AMAZING FLAPJACKS

One of my Wild Ginger Running monthly supporters, Darren, brings these incredible home-made flapjacks with him whenever we have a meet-up. They're deliciously tasty and energy-boosting towards the end of a long, hilly run.

MAKE IT

Preheat the oven to 220°C/190°C fan/gas mark 7. Melt 200g (8oz) butter, 200g (8oz) golden caster sugar and 80g (3^1/$_5$ oz) golden syrup in a pan. Gradually stir in 250g (10oz) oats. Mix in 2 large tbsp crunchy peanut butter. Pour into an 18cm (7in) square baking tin lined with baking paper. Bake for 14 minutes, then remove from the oven and leave to cool in the tin. Melt 150g (6oz) chocolate, then spread over the cooked flapjack. Leave to set. Cut into bite-sized pieces and pop them in a ziplock bag.

VARY IT

You can of course leave off the chocolate (this is a good idea in hot weather or you'll end up in a mess). You can also add all sorts of things to the mixture: dried cranberries or raisins, chopped dried ready-to-eat apricots, chopped nuts or some seeds – whatever you fancy.

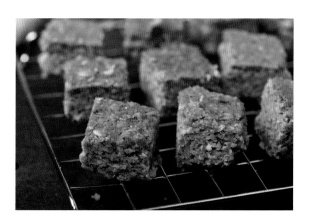

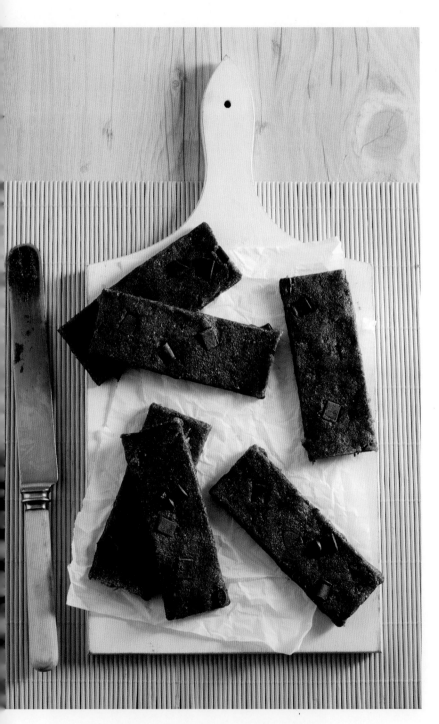

ANITA BEAN'S DARK CHOC CHIP ENERGY BARS

These are so easy – there is no cooking involved, simply mixing. *The Runner's Cookbook* author Anita Bean says: 'Cocoa and dark chocolate chips are rich in polyphenols, which help increase oxygen delivery to muscles during endurance exercise.'

MAKE IT

Whizz up 150g (6oz) Medjool dates, 100g (4oz) dried ready-to-eat apricots, 125g (5oz) raw almonds, 1 tbsp cocoa powder and 1 tsp ground cinnamon in a food processor until it sticks together. Add 25g (1oz) choc chips and pulse until it feels like stiff cookie dough. Line a tin with cling film and press in the mixture, then cut into slices. Keep refrigerated for up to a week or freeze for up to three months.

VARY IT

You can vary the nuts and dried fruit to create other flavour combos. Cashews are great as they are soft and whizz up easily, and soft prunes make a good alternative to apricots.

CRISPS

These are very easy to find in shops and are a great source of salty, fatty fuel for long runs. I often use the empty crisp packet as a bin bag for other snack wrappers as it tends to be hardy and roomy.

CHEESE

For longer runs, a salty, creamy taste is good, so chunks of strong Cheddar that isn't too crumbly work well. You can buy fun-sized packs with each chunk wrapped in plastic already, or go for the more eco-friendly method of chopping your own into an old crisp packet.

BABY POTATOES

Pre-cooked and bagged up with a little salt, these are delicious and filling when eaten with a chunk of cheese. Pop them into your pocket warm on winter runs for a hot water bottle effect for the first half hour to help get you out of the door.

MINI PORK PIES AND MINI SCOTCH EGGS

Widely available at most supermarkets, this easy-to-carry, ready-to-eat, bite-sized picnic food is perfect for a savoury moving buffet. Consume within a couple of hours if the weather is warm, or it is possible to freeze them and let them defrost for a couple of hours if you're out for a really long run in very hot weather.

VEGGIE BURGERS

Once I had a veggie burger left over from dinner the night before so I wrapped it up and took it with me – it was delicious, if a little crumbly, but if you squash it together more before cooking then that can help!

PIZZA

Pimp up a cheese and tomato pizza with your favourite topping (mushroom, spinach and feta is good!), cook as per the packet instructions, leave to cool, fold in half (to keep the filling inside), slice and bag one or two up for your run.

VEGAN CHEESE THINS

Two slices of vegan cheese in a bread 'thin' makes an easy-to-eat, tasty savoury snack for a long run.

CREAM CHEESE CROISSANT

These squash down easily in cling film (or a reused plastic bag) and you can easily make them vegan, with alternatives for both products available.

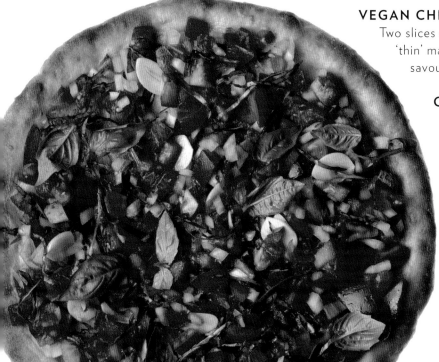

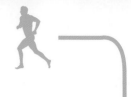

HYDRATION

Drinking is just as important as eating, because when you start to warm up on a run (and have taken off as many layers as possible) losing fluid through sweat is your body's best way of cooling down. It's even more important in hot climates, where you will be losing more fluid and salts through sweat, and for people who naturally sweat more than others. Hydration is often overlooked, but dehydration and overhydration can be at best detrimental to your performance and at worst life-threatening. Being properly hydrated also speeds up your recovery. There are no set rules on how much you should drink and when to drink as it varies so much from person to person, weather conditions and climate, but here are the basic guidelines.

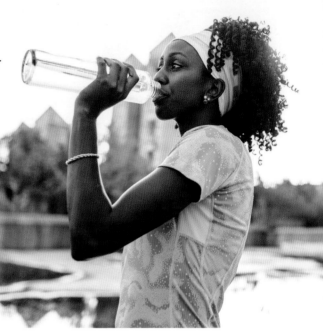

STAY HYDRATED
Take small sips of fluid often throughout the day so you start every run well hydrated. Take small sips throughout runs of more than 60–90 minutes or in hotter weather or climates. Drink to thirst and ask yourself at regular intervals, 'Am I thirsty?' If in doubt, take a few small sips. Don't let yourself get thirsty to the point where you want to grab water and gulp it down like you've been lost in the desert – your kidneys can only cope with so much water at a time so a lot of this will end up in your bladder. Use electrolytes

(see opposite) to combat the salts lost through sweating. Have a drink ready for when you've finished your run and drink it steadily to thirst.

DANGEROUS OVERHYDRATION
The advice used to be to drink before you were thirsty, but drinking really excessive amounts of water can cause a very dangerous condition called hyponatraemia. This is where excess water has caused the sodium (salt) concentration in the blood to lower to a critical level. Symptoms include stomach ache, dizziness, nausea, bloating

and, in very extreme cases, total collapse and death. Don't worry though, hyponatraemia is extremely rare and you are highly unlikely to get it if you drink according to the guidelines here.

DEHYDRATION

Dehydration (when you haven't drunk enough water) is much more common and mild dehydration is not usually dangerous but can have a detrimental impact on your performance and recovery. Symptoms include a dry mouth, headache, only being able to produce small amounts of darker yellow urine, thirst, unusual fatigue and lack of energy, feeling too hot, feeling sick and dizziness.

TEST YOUR WEE

Your urine should be the colour of pale straw if you're properly hydrated. If it is more orange or dark orange, drink a little more.

ALCOHOL...?

Alcohol is a diuretic, so it makes you need to wee more, which rids you of water and electrolytes (mineral salts, such as sodium, chloride, potassium and magnesium). This is obviously not the best thing before, during or after a run or race. However, I have spoken to athletes who drink a glass of red wine to settle nerves and aid sleep before a big race, there are whole marathons with wine stops en route and many runners enjoy celebrating with a beer. If you run for fun rather than peak performance, alcohol is fine in moderation, but I would recommend rehydrating first with a pint of water, squash or orange juice mixed with soda water or lemonade (if you want a seriously sugary hit) and making every other drink a soft drink or water.

'Doing short, three to four hour races, the only thing I'd have was my little bottle of home-made salt and glucose drink, that'd get us round.'

Joss Naylor, legendary Lake District fell runner

DIY ELECTROLYTE DRINK

Use this for shorter runs of 60–90 minutes as you lose electrolytes when you sweat (see p. 190). However, you don't need any added energy from sugar. You can buy electrolyte tablets, powders and ready-made drinks, but here's a simple recipe to make your own.

MAKE IT

Mix up your favourite flavour of sugar-free squash in a 500ml (17fl oz) water bottle, then add a pinch of table salt.

DIY ISOTONIC DRINK

Ideal for runs over two hours long in hot, humid conditions, isotonic drinks have the same concentrations of salt and sugar as your blood, meaning they are rapidly absorbed, quickly help maintain blood sugar levels and increase endurance. You can also find them as ready-made drinks in shops, but making your own works well too. Add a touch more salt if you sweat excessively or if it's very hot.

MAKE IT

Mix up your favourite flavour of sugar-free squash in a 500ml (17fl oz) water bottle, then add 2 pinches of table salt and 2 tsp sugar.

DIY ENERGY DRINK

Great for runs over two to three hours long, energy drinks use a blend of simple carbohydrates (sugars), often around 30–45g per 500ml water (1^1/$_4$–1^3/$_4$ oz per 17fl oz water). Many shop-bought drinks are packed with sugar so adding a pinch of salt to them works, and there are dedicated sports energy drinks too. Using normal table sugar is fine as this is scientifically known as sucrose – a blend of glucose and fructose that is easily absorbed during running.

MAKE IT

Mix up your favourite flavour of sugar-free squash in a 500ml (17fl oz) water bottle, then add 2 pinches of table salt and 90g (3^1/$_2$ oz) sucrose (table sugar). Shake well.

ANITA BEAN'S DIY CHERRY RECOVERY DRINK

Perfect for post-run rehydration, ideally within the first two hours afterwards, recovery drinks contain the optimum ratio of carbs to protein (3:1) for a swift recovery. They usually contain 20–60g (^{4}/$_5$–2^1/$_2$ oz) carbs (sugars) and 10–20g (^{2}/$_5$–^{4}/$_5$ oz) protein – often whey, casein or soy. It's great to drink if you won't be eating for a while after your run or race. Semi-skimmed milk provides an excellent mix of carbs and protein, but there are options for vegans too. This one, by sports nutritionist Anita Bean, contains cherries, which she says: 'are rich in anthocyanins that help reduce inflammation and promote recovery, while the other ingredients replenish your carbs, electrolytes and protein.'

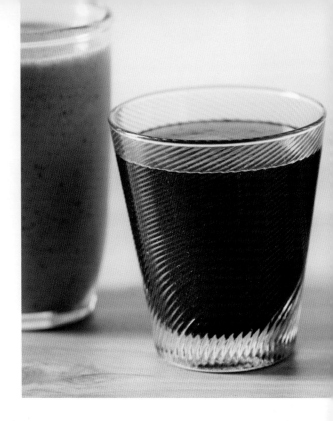

MAKE IT

Blitz 125ml (4^1/$_4$fl oz) milk or plain yoghurt (or a combination), 125ml (4^1/$_4$fl oz) water, 125g (5oz) frozen, pitted cherries, 1 sliced banana and 2 tsp honey in a blender or smoothie maker until smooth. Pour into a glass and drink immediately, or it will keep in the fridge for up to two days.

VARY IT

You can of course use plant-based milk and yoghurt. Experiment with other dark red fruits, such as frozen mixed berries, though you may need to adjust the sweetness to taste.

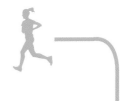

RECOVERY SNACKS

Protein and carbohydrate-rich snacks will help you recover quickly, replenishing your muscles' stores of glycogen and repairing damaged fibres. Scientists agree that a ratio of 3:1 carbs to protein is optimal and it's best to eat such food within two hours of finishing running (or any intense exercise) as this is when your body is most receptive. This could be a full meal, in which case you don't need these snacks. However, these six snacks do come in handy if dinner's not for a while after your run or race. To drink your recovery in the form of a smoothie, see the cherry recovery drink recipe on the previous page.

1 GREEK YOGHURT

Easy to grab from the shops and a food that slides down super easily after a run, a 125g (5oz) pot packs a delicious protein-rich punch.

2 HARD-BOILED EGG

Packed with protein to fill your belly and easy to transport, eggs are a deliciously healthy recovery snack you can pre-prepare and take anywhere if it's not too hot.

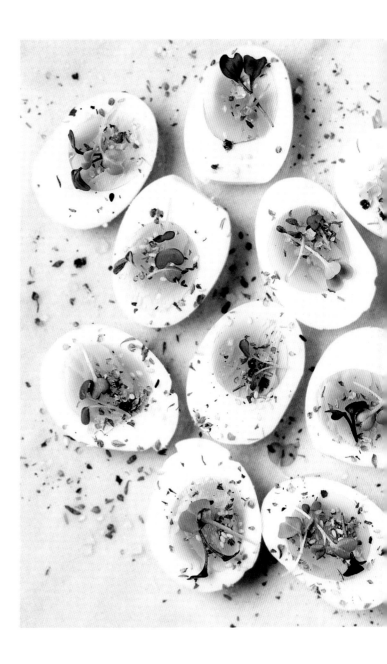

3 TUNA

If you buy a tin with a ring pull on it then tuna becomes a light, portable recovery snack that lasts a long time. It can be slightly dry on its own though, so you may prefer to buy one in healthy olive oil, which moistens it nicely, or in a pouch with mayo already added.

4 TRAIL MIX

Nuts and dried fruit are the perfect source of delicious healthy protein, quick-release carbs and healthy fats to speed up your recovery. Experiment with different types and mix up the combinations to keep life exciting.

5 CHOCOLATE MILK

Easy to find in the shops, and available made with milk alternatives, this is also a cinch to make.

MAKE IT

Simply measure out 150ml (5fl oz) milk, add it dash by dash to 1^1/$_2$ tsp cocoa powder and 1 tsp icing sugar, stirring to make a paste, then thin it out slowly with more milk.

VARY IT

Swap the cocoa and sugar for a flavoured protein powder – strawberry, chocolate and vanilla are especially palatable. You can use any type of milk, though cow's milk is best for helping to repair micro-tears in the muscles (see p. 122)

6 ANITA BEAN'S CINNAMON CRANBERRY GRANOLA BARS

Delicious and easy to make, *The Runner's Cookbook* author Anita Bean says: 'These bars contain the ideal balance of carbohydrate and protein plus essential fats and antioxidant nutrients (especially cranberries with their high polyphenol content) to aid muscle repair.'

MAKE IT

Preheat the oven to 190°C/170°C fan/gas mark 5. Line a 23cm (9in) square baking tin with baking paper. Heat 200g (7oz) dried dates in a small saucepan with 4 tbsp water for five minutes or until soft. Add 75g (3oz) honey and mix until smooth. Pour into a large bowl and mix in ^{1}/$_2$ tsp ground cinnamon, 125g (5oz) oats, 100g (4oz) chopped walnuts, 100g (4oz) mixed seeds and 50g (2oz) dried cranberries. Press the mixture into the tin, bake for 20 minutes or until firm, leave to cool, then slice into 12 pieces. Keep in a tin for up to a week.

VARY IT

Vary the fruits, nuts and seeds according to what you like and have to hand.

SPORTS NUTRITION PRODUCTS

Sports nutrition products such as gels, energy bars and energy drink powders are often promoted as wonder performance-enhancing fuel that you must not miss. And yes, many contain nutritious ingredients, energy and protein to boost performance and recovery, but there is nothing in them that you cannot get from a healthy, balanced diet at a fraction at the price. However, sports nutrition products do have the advantage of being a very convenient source of light, packable, easily opened, ingested and digested nutrition with a long storage date.

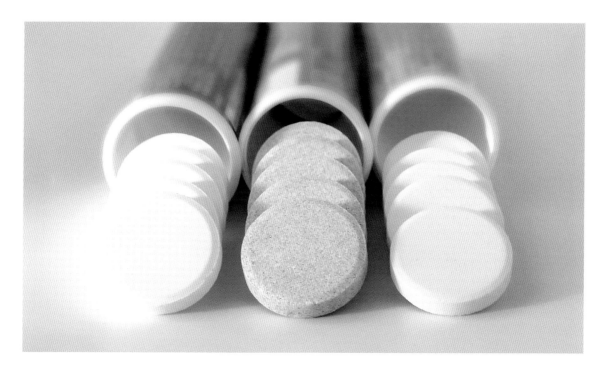

GELS

These are handy, easy-to-open, easy-to-eat tubes of high-energy (high-carbohydrate) gel with a huge variety of flavours and various viscosities, ranging from gloopy to ganache.

They're often the go-to fuel for fast races over 60–90 minutes long, and they range in size and shape but are usually 30–60ml (1–2fl oz). Smaller is sometimes better as it's sticky and difficult to store an opened gel if you only want to consume half at a time. Some gels contain more water than others and the drier they are the more water you may need to consume with them in order to avoid digestion issues. Some people find their stomachs don't get on so well with gels, but others, especially elite athletes working at flat-out paces, find them the perfect way to ingest energy for races up to six to seven hours long. Some gels also contain caffeine to boost performance and beat fatigue.

BARS

Super convenient to pop in your running pack or pocket, energy and/or protein bars are a very popular choice, especially on longer, slower runs when you have the time, energy and enough saliva to chew. They usually range from 40–60g ($1^1/_2$–$2^1/_2$ oz) and they are easier than gels if you want to take a mouthful at a time and feel more substantial, like real food. Although their main aim is to fill you with quick-release energy in the form of sugar, some bars contain more natural ingredients than others, so look for ones made of real food that you recognise, such as dried fruits, oats, nuts and seeds.

CHEWS/BEANS

Bridging the gap between sloppy gels and solid bars, chews (and maybe also beans) are the sports nutrition industry's version of the humble Jelly Babies – easy-to-eat sweets packed with energy. The advantage of these versus normal sweets is that rather than being made from pure glucose they often use a combination of different sugars, such as maltodextrin, sucrose and fructose, which have different absorption rates, so you should get less of a sugar spike and be able to absorb more.

ELECTROLYTES

These are usually sold in tablet form so you can take a couple on a run to add to your water bottle when you refill it. You lose electrolytes (mineral salts, such as sodium, chloride, potassium and magnesium) when you sweat and it's vital to replace them because they help control fluid balance, muscle contraction and energy production. If you sweat heavily then you may need more electrolytes to prevent cramps, dehydration and a drop in performance, so it may be worth having a sweat test analysis (a test that measures the amount of chloride in your sweat) for runners to gauge your exact electrolyte needs.

POWDERS

Powders are a particularly handy and portable way to add electrolytes, carbs, protein or a combination of these to drinks before, after or during a run. They are often sold in bulk in large containers and come in many different-flavoured varieties, from 'flavourless' to chocolate to tropical fruit.

SPORTS DRINKS

Ready-made sports drinks come in various types, including low-calorie electrolyte, isotonic and energy. Electrolyte-only drinks don't contain any energy – they replace the salts you lose from sweating (see above). Isotonic drinks have the same concentrations of salt and sugar as your bodily fluids so they help maintain blood sugar levels and increase endurance. Energy drinks contain sugar (usually glucose, maltodextrin and fructose) and provide more energy.

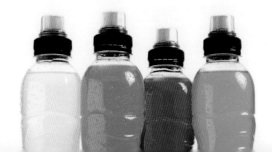

DO YOU NEED SPORTS SUPPLEMENTS?

These are designed to enhance performance using higher doses of boosters such as creatine, caffeine and nitrate than would normally be found in foods. Sports nutritionist Anita Bean, author of *The Runner's Cookbook,* says: 'These products promise you'll run faster and recover quicker, but in truth, you can get everything you need for this from real food. There is also no guarantee that all these products are free from banned substances so check www.informed-sport.com for trusted brands. However, below I list some natural performance enhancers that have been scientifically proven to work effectively. Always experiment carefully with these, in training rather than race day, to find the dose and timing that works best for you.'

Natural sports supplements

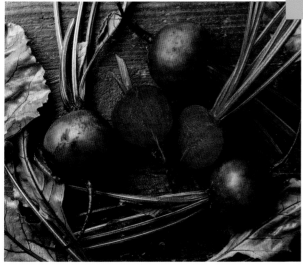

CHERRY FOR RECOVERY

The antioxidants in Montmorency cherries may reduce the inflammation associated with delayed onset muscle soreness (DOMS) and promote recovery. Try drinking 30ml (1fl oz) Montmorency sour cherry juice four to five days before and two days after long races.

CAFFEINE FOR PERFORMANCE

This is a well-known stimulant that blocks the brain chemical adenosine that normally makes you feel tired, increasing alertness and concentration and lowering perceived effort so exercise feels easier. The caffeine in coffee is not regulated or stated so it can vary cup to cup. It will boost your performance pre-race for short races, but for longer races or more of a scientific trial of your needs, try a gel containing 60–180mg caffeine. Take it 30–45 minutes before you need it, before a short race or towards the end of a longer one. It can cause an upset stomach or an urge to empty the bowels in some though, so try caffeine in training before a race.

BEETROOT FOR ENDURANCE

The nitrate in beetroots (converted to nitric oxide in the body) may improve endurance and efficiency by helping to dilate blood vessels, increase blood flow and allow more blood to reach the muscles faster. Try beetroot loading three to seven days before a big race, or take one or two 70ml (2.4fl oz) shots of concentrated beetroot juice two to three hours before short races.

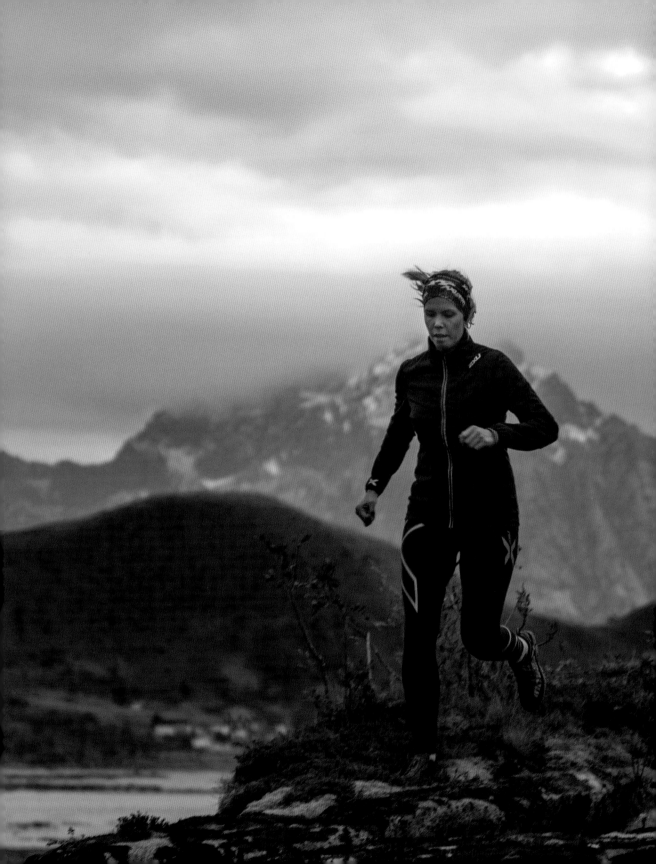

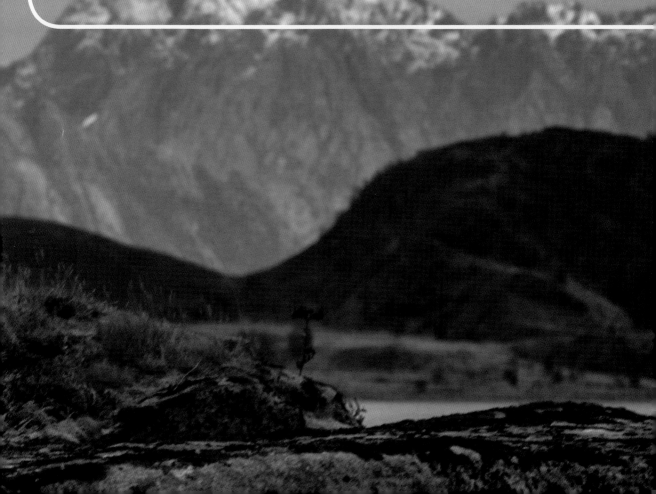

7

RACES AND CHALLENGES

One of the most fantastic aspects of trail and ultra running is that races and challenges can take you all over the country, all over the world even – it's a great way to explore within the safety and camaraderie of an organised event.

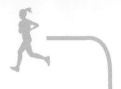

YOUR FIRST TRAIL RACE

There are so many fantastic trail races and running festivals in beautiful locations all over the UK. And unlike road races, where the emphasis is on speed, split times and personal bests, trail races with generous cut-off times are a safe and exciting way to see a new area on a waymarked, marshalled course without having to map read. Double-check the navigation level required in the race details, but most trail races are waymarked or follow clear National Trail signage. This means that plenty of trail races are great for newcomers. Here are my experiences and recommendations.

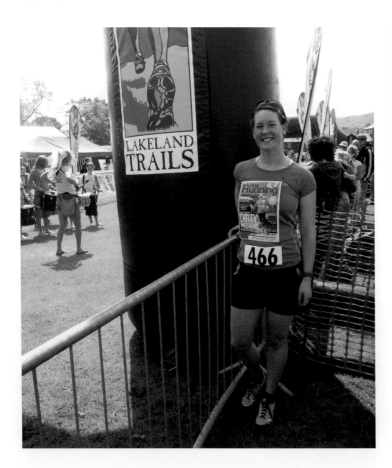

'The best way to believe in yourself is to do things that are difficult and scary! Challenge yourself, change your mindset, change your life.'

Sophie Radcliffe,
adventurer and speaker

FIND A RACE NEAR YOU

I use SiEntries and Find a Race as they have lots of great races listed with useful filter options. Check out the Wild Ginger Running Recommended Races YouTube playlist for more of my favourites.

MY FIRST TRAIL RACE

My first ever trail race was the Lakeland Trails Coniston 15k in the Lake District. After a long drive with endless delays, I got there by the skin of my teeth and changed in my car with 10 minutes to spare. I rushed to the registration tent and just about pinned my race number on when the starting gun fired. It was a cool, October day and as a hill walker, I hadn't appreciated how hot I'd get after only five minutes' running uphill. Other runners clad in shorts and T-shirts streamed past as I took off my windproof, long-sleeved base layer, gloves and hat! I didn't have a pack so I tied them round my waist and put the accessories in my pockets, where they banged around annoyingly for the whole race. It was hard work, but I was pleased I wasn't alone in walking breathlessly up the hills. Then came the views. Stupendous vistas across Coniston Water, the Old Man of Coniston topped with clouds, and waterfalls cascading through the former copper mines. It was breathtaking. I didn't want it to end.

FROM ROAD TO TRAIL RACES

'We were terrified on the start line of our first trail race, convinced we couldn't complete the distance. After over a decade of road running races including a marathon, my sister and I entered a 100k ultra for a new challenge! Realising this was a very long way, we found a shorter trail race with no cut-off times as we were worried about our pace. We emailed the organisers and they reassured us, so we lined up with scarily fit-looking runners and, helped by the race team, we finished last at 1a.m. They were all there to applaud us and share a beer. Best event ever.'

CLARE CARTER, BRISTOL

But down we ran, along wide, twisting trails, never too rocky to put the brakes on. We flew down to a glorious field finish cheered on by friends, faster runners, high-fiving kids, excited dogs and an energetic drumming band. After a chat with other runners and an ice cream I forgot the initial sweaty slog and decided to book a whole-series season ticket for the next year!

TOP 10 TIPS FOR YOUR FIRST TRAIL RACE

1 PREPARE RIGHT

As well as the obvious training that's involved with the distance you've chosen, make sure you get on the race website and read the details too. The race may well have a list of mandatory kit you need to take, which you might need time to beg, steal or borrow, there might be important info about parking and food availability, and registration might be a little walk from the start. Get this prep right to avoid any unnecessary stress on race morning.

2 LAY OUT YOUR KIT

You might have seen social media posts from other runners with their kit laid out on the floor the night before an event, sometimes with their race number already safely pinned to their top if it has been pre-sent or they registered that evening. This is a great way to get organised and make sure you have everything so you can simply get up and hop into your running gear with zero palaver. The gear section in chapter 5 will help you with this part too.

3 PLAN YOUR BREAKFAST

Make sure you know what time your race starts and plan to eat a small meal at least two hours beforehand. If you can, get it ready the night before: for example, put your porridge in a bowl ready for the milk or leave a loaf of bread near the toaster with a plate, knife, peanut butter and jam ready beside it. This all cuts down on brainwork pre-race so you feel fully prepared and ready. There's also a race fuel timeline on pp. 176-177.

4 GET THERE EARLY

Plan to arrive at your race at least an hour before the start, more if you can as you need time to park, find registration, register, sort out your race number, warm up and pop back to the car to ditch warm layers or leave it with friends or family. There may also be a map of the route and gradient profile so you can check out where the main climbs are if you haven't already seen this online.

5 WARM UP

About 20 minutes before the race start, do the warm-up on pp. 60-62, wearing joggers and a warm top if it's cold. If you feel like taking a layer of clothing off at the end of your warm-up, you've done it right! Be bold, start cold. I was a wimp at the start of my first trail races and wore lots of layers, only to have to slow down and tie them all round my waist at the first hill!

6 START SLOWLY

No one wants to hear this, but if you only do ONE thing in this list, make it this! It's so, so easy to set off at breakneck speed, spurred on by the other runners around you, feeling like you could run this fast all day. It might take a few races before you can rein in this temptation, but if you start off steadily for the first 10 minutes, ease into a rhythmical pace and save your big effort until you're a couple of miles from the end, you'll actually do better and find it a whole lot easier too. Plus there's the mental boost of running past everyone who started off too fast!

7 WALK THE HILLS

If the gradient ahead starts to rear up, run steadily as far as you can until you feel your breath start to get out of control. Then start walking briskly instead (some people call this power hiking as it sounds cooler). Another sign that the hill is too steep to run is that others around you will also be walking, or that you are walking as fast as some others are running!

8 SMILE!

Remember to look at all the gorgeous views and smile. This is why you run, isn't it? Not just for fitness and performance, but also to take yourself to beautiful places and surround yourself with like-minded, friendly people. You might even exchange a few words with the runners around you if you can spare the breath. It all makes for a memorable race experience.

9 FINISH STRONG

With a couple of miles to go (if you've managed numbers 6 and 7!), you might have a surge in energy as you realise how close you are to finishing your first ever trail race. Harness this and pick up the pace slightly, enjoying bounding along, especially as it's hopefully all downhill

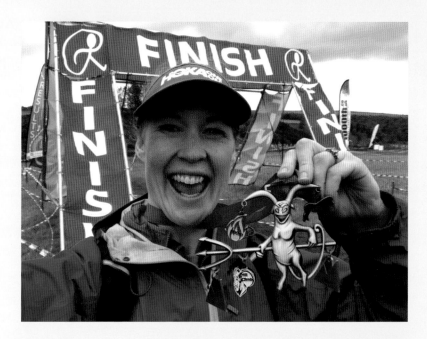

from here. Keep a little bit back, saving your final powerful sprint for the last 100m (110 yards) across the finish line to the roar of the crowd, inspiring family or friends who are watching you.

10 TREAT YOURSELF!

It's treat time! Follow the sensible recovery advice on pp. 76–77, but mainly now is the time to reward yourself for your amazing efforts on your first ever trail race. Treat yourself to that piece of gear you've been ogling for ages, an ice cream, a beer, or all three if you're feeling flush. Relax and enjoy the race atmosphere, chat to fellow runners you met on the course and wear that medal or T-shirt with pride. You've earned it.

1 PARKRUN 5K, EVERYWHERE, EVERY SATURDAY

parkrun is a fantastic way to start running off-road as none of them are on roads! They can be on tarmac though, so if allowed, run on any grass or gravel next to the course to make it a trail.

2 LAKELAND TRAILS, LAKE DISTRICT

Family-friendly, well-marked trail runs and walks in the beautiful Lake District mountainside throughout the year, with distances such as 5km (3.1 miles), 10km (6.2 miles), 15km (9.3 miles), 18km (11.2 miles), 23km (14.3 miles) and beyond.

3 ENDURANCELIFE RACES

Well-signposted 10k, half marathon, marathon and ultra distance trail races all over the UK, mainly on stunning coastal trails from Cornwall to Northumberland.

4 NATIONAL TRUST 10

Free, monthly, untimed 10k trail runs through National Trust woodland paths starting at 9a.m. on various dates and locations throughout the UK.

5 MAVERICK RACES

Exciting night races and original day races from 5km (3.1 miles) to 50km (31 miles) in England and Wales with many in the south and just outside London.

6 ENDURE24

Known as 'Glastonbury for runners', gather your trail running friends for a 24-hour team camp-out and relay race around an undulating 8km (5-mile) loop in Reading or Leeds.

7 RUN. COED Y BRENIN

Year-round running and night running from 5k to marathon on the specially created trails in Coed y Brenin Forest Park, Snowdonia.

TRAIL HACK

BEAT POST-RACE BLUES

When you've been focusing on preparing for a big trail race, once it's over it's not unusual to feel lost and depressed with all the excitement suddenly gone. Beat these post-race blues by picking another goal to get excited about. It might be another trail race or your own running challenge, but the goal doesn't have to even be running related. Maybe it's a family holiday or a skills course, or making a patchwork quilt out of your old race T-shirts. Whatever it is, choose something that excites and re-energises you.

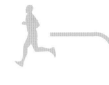

MY FAVOURITE TRAIL RACES

During my seven years editing *Trail Running* magazine I had the great pleasure to run so many brilliant trail races all over the world. Here are my absolute favourites.

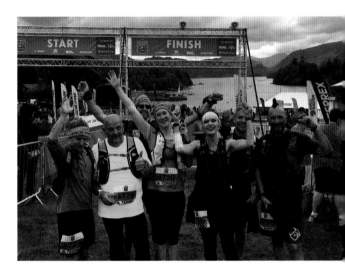

DEAD SEA HALF MARATHON, ISRAEL, FEBRUARY

Super-easy running on a wide, flat, gritty path, fantastic for beginners; on the edge of the Dead Sea. It was unreal to run past perfectly circular salt islands and there's jaw-dropping trail running in the nearby desert wadis if you can stay longer. Also 10k and marathon options.

MANX MOUNTAIN MARATHON, ISLE OF MAN, APRIL

I have such fond memories of this unbelievably stunning 30-mile (48.3km) mountain and coastal trail from Ramsey to Port Erin, including the island's highest mountain, Snaefell. Also a half marathon option.

KESWICK MOUNTAIN FESTIVAL 25K, LAKE DISTRICT, MAY

I've done this race about five times now with my local running club and Wild Ginger Running channel Patreons and it's an absolutely beautiful, rocky-pathed circuit of Derwent Water with testing climbs, wonderful descents and awesome views. Also 5k, 10k and ultra.

NENE VALLEY TRAIL RACES, NORTHAMPTONSHIRE, JUNE

Who knew there were beautiful trails in the Midlands? OK, I'm biased as I organise this race with two other trail-loving ladies from my local club, Stamford Striders, but we have a super 10- or 20-miler (16km or 32km) along disused railway lines, through undulating fields past rivers and picturesque, ancient stone villages.

PEAK SKYLINE, PEAK DISTRICT, AUGUST

I absolutely loved this hilly but mostly runnable tour of this area's pointiest summits, including the beautifully boulder-edged Roaches and Shutlingsloe, the Matterhorn of the Peak District. It's just over a marathon at 30 miles (48.3km), but they have a 14.5-mile (23.3km) race too.

ICEBUG XPERIENCE, SWEDEN, SEPTEMBER

This is an absolutely fantastic three-day event on Bohuslän's undulating coast in west Sweden. With distances ranging from 22km (13.7 miles) to 29km (18 miles), there's plenty of time to soak up the sea, lake and forest views, refuel on cinnamon buns at the many checkpoints and sample delicious local food each evening.

ENNERDALE TRAIL RUN, LAKE DISTRICT, OCTOBER

The 25k is a fantastic whole loop of Ennerdale Water, setting out on an easy wide path through forest and returning along a tricky, rocky trail. I hopped in the lake afterwards to cool my legs down and was thrilled to interview Joss Naylor, who was presenting the prizes. There is also a 10k option.

OTHER EXCITING TRAIL EVENTS

NIGHT RUNNING

Running in the dark is exhilarating – it truly feels like you're flying through crisp darkness under starry skies. Get a head torch with 200+ lumens for enough light to see the trails (see p. 153), take it easy if you can't see clearly what you're running over and carry an extra layer as it's always colder at night.

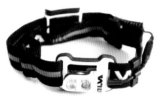

TRY IT!
Kielder Dark Skies Run Series, Northumberland, March.
Run 10km (6.2 miles), 14 miles (22.5km) or 26 miles (41.8km) after sunset around Kielder reservoir and Dark Sky Park, lit by twinkling starlight and your fellow competitors' head torches.

NAVIGATION EVENTS

Map reading while running adds another dimension to your new fave sport, not to mention another string to your bow. Follow the navigation tips on p. 52, but the best advice is to slow down until you know exactly where you are going!

TRY IT!
OMM (Original Mountain Marathon) Lite, May.
You can do this two-day event solo or in pairs, navigating round Cannock Chase to as many checkpoints as you can in a set timeframe. Each has a different score and the aim is to get as many points as possible without being late back.

TRAIL RUNNING FESTIVALS

Weekend running festivals with races or guided runs and talks, films and/or music in the evening are a fantastic way to hang out with like-minded people, learn new things and explore a beautiful new location.

TRY IT!
Keswick Mountain Festival, RunFestRun, Love Trails Festival, Top of the Gorge, South West Outdoor Festival, Something Wild Trail Running Festival, Runstock and Big Running Weekend. All of the above are fantastic.

TRAIL RUNNING TRAINING CAMPS

These are the ultimate way to improve your off-road running technique and skills with expert tuition in a small, friendly and supportive group in a beautiful trail location.

TRY IT!
Wild Ginger Running Training Camp.
This is an information-packed long weekend for beginner to intermediate level, including hill techniques, strength work, nutrition, navigation, night running, gear testing, expert talks and exclusive films.

CREATE YOUR OWN CHALLENGE

Explore a new place at your own pace, set yourself a speed challenge on a local hill or break down a long-distance race or trail into a more manageable weekend or multi-day running holiday.

TRY IT!
Raad ny Foillan coastal path, Isle of Man.
This 100-mile (160km) path fits neatly into a six-day run with distances from 13–24 miles (21–38.6km) each day, along hilly sea cliff paths at seabird height and beach running past seals.

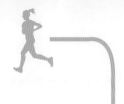

TRAIL RACES OVERSEAS

Trail races are a fantastic way to see the world and explore foreign lands within the safety net of a well-organised event. Here are a dozen of the world's best.

1 SIERRE-ZINAL, SWITZERLAND, AUGUST

One of the oldest and most scenic mountain races in Europe, 5200 competitors run 31km (19.3 miles) through the Valais Alps in Switzerland around five 4000m (13,123ft) summits with 2200m (7218ft) of ascent.

2 ROSA RUN, RUSSIA, MAY

A four-day running festival in Sochi, in the mountains, with a vertical kilometre and two trail runs, one 8km (5 miles) and one 26km (16.2 miles), along tree-lined trails with snow-capped summit views.

3 STRANDA FJORD TRAIL RACE, NORWAY, AUGUST

Choose from 25km (155 miles) or 48km (30 miles) distances through incredible mountain and fjord scenery with jaw-dropping views, long climbs and descents and some rocky sections underfoot.

4 BIG FIVE MARATHON AND HALF MARATHON, SOUTH AFRICA, JUNE

Multi-terrain races beside zebra, giraffes and antelopes and possibly even lions (time for a personal best?) on trails, stony tracks and dirt roads in the African Savannah.

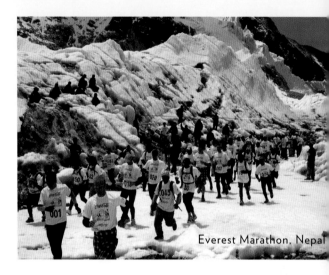
Everest Marathon, Nepal

5 ORIGINAL EVEREST MARATHON (OMM), NEPAL, DECEMBER

The Guinness World Records' highest marathon in the world! Reaching the start line is a challenge in itself – a 15-day trek up to Everest Base Camp at 5184m (17,000ft) above sea level before your 26-mile (41.8km) run along narrow trails and high wire suspension bridges.

6 AUSTRALIAN OUTBACK MARATHON, AUSTRALIA, JULY

Stunning views of the iconic red sandstone Uluru (Ayers Rock) and Kata Tjuta (the Olgas) for all levels of runner with 6km (3.7km), 10km (6.2-mile), half marathon and marathon options.

7 TARAWERA ULTRAMARATHON, NEW ZEALAND, FEBRUARY

The country's most famous 100-mile (160km) endurance run also has 21.1km (13.1-mile) and

50km (31-mile) races, starting at a steaming geyser with a route through redwood forest and beside vibrant blue and green lakes.

8 PIKES PEAK MARATHON, USA, AUGUST

An iconic race once run by UK fell running legend Joss Naylor, in mountainous Colorado up to the 4302m (14,114ft) summit of the beautiful Pikes Peak and back down. You can also do the Ascent race, a half marathon uphill all the way to the top!

9 INCA TRAIL MARATHON, SOUTH AMERICA, JUNE AND AUGUST

Billed as 'The most difficult marathon in the world', following the original stone-stepped and narrow trail route to the incredible lost Inca city of Machu Picchu.

10 FUJI MOUNTAIN RACE, JAPAN, JULY

Clamber up through dense forest and then out onto shifting volcanic stones and grit all the way to the summit of Mount Fuji on this 21.1km (13.1-mile) race, the country's highest peak at 3776m (12,388ft).

11 ICELAND VOLCANO MARATHON, ICELAND, JULY

Run 26 miles (41.8km) beside geysers, glaciers and strangely shaped lava rocks on dirt tracks and black volcano sand in this hotbed of geothermal activity.

12 ANTARCTIC ICE MARATHON, ANTARCTICA, DECEMBER

Try the world's most southerly marathon, running across vast plains of pure white snow and ice a few hundred miles from the South Pole, at the foot of the Ellsworth Mountains.

TRAIL HACK

OFFSET YOUR CARBON

As trail runners, we know how important it is to protect the wilderness that we love to run in, so consider offsetting the environmental impact of your travel to overseas races by using an online carbon calculator and donating this small amount to a reputable carbon offset company funding renewable energy projects. https://projectwren.com/

MY STORY

IT DOESN'T HAVE TO BE A RACE

'I was a road runner with no experience in trail running but I was looking for a challenge, so I signed up for a Tracks and Trails trail running camp in Chamonix, France, in 2016 and then a trail running trip in 2018. I learned how to tackle technical descents, using poles, running in snow, nutrition, heart rate monitoring and pacing. Little did I know I would fall in love with trail running and eventually complete the 42km [26-mile] Mont Blanc Marathon in 2019!'

JULIANNE CIRENZA, LONDON

THE WORLD'S MOST FAMOUS RACES

Once you dip your toe into the trail running world, you'll find there are certain iconic off-road races that have become famous enough even for non-runners to know about. They tend to be towards the more extreme end, both in distance and difficulty, and some definitely aren't trail races, but I wanted to include them here as they're exciting to follow. You might want to attempt one of these one day, or maybe you think they're utterly barmy! There's no pressure either way – running them, following them on social media, crewing others and spectating are all fantastic ways to get involved with these classic, unforgettable events.

WESTERN STATES ENDURANCE RUN, USA

This highly sought-after race in Squaw Valley, California claims to be the world's oldest 100-mile (160km) race and it has the best story. The race started off as the Tevis Cup 100-mile (160km) one-day trail ride in 1955 to prove that horses could still cover that distance in 24 hours. Gordy Ainsleigh impressed everyone by completing it bareback in 1971. It became the most important event in Gordy's year, but in 1974, his horse became lame. He didn't want to miss out, so he ran it, proving that humans could also run 100 miles (160km) in one day. Three years later, the first official Western States Endurance Run took place with three men finishing. Now, so many people want to enter there's a lottery system for the 369 places the race organisers are legally allowed in this wilderness area. Hardrock 100 and Leadville Trail 100 are also very famous ultras in the USA.

ULTRA-TRAIL DU MONT-BLANC (UTMB), FRANCE

The Ultra-Trail du Mont-Blanc is arguably the Olympics of trail running, one of the world's biggest races with a stacked field of the best athletes from across the globe. This 106-mile (170km) trail run with a whopping 10,000m (32,808ft) ascent starts in the French mountain town of Chamonix on the last weekend in August. The route passes through Italy and Switzerland on its circumnavigation of the highest mountain in the Alps, Mont Blanc, through Courmayeur and Champex-Lac before the final push back to Chamonix, where crowds of thousands clang cow bells and cheer each finisher as if they were the winner. Spectating, crewing or racing is an experience not to be missed for every trail runner.

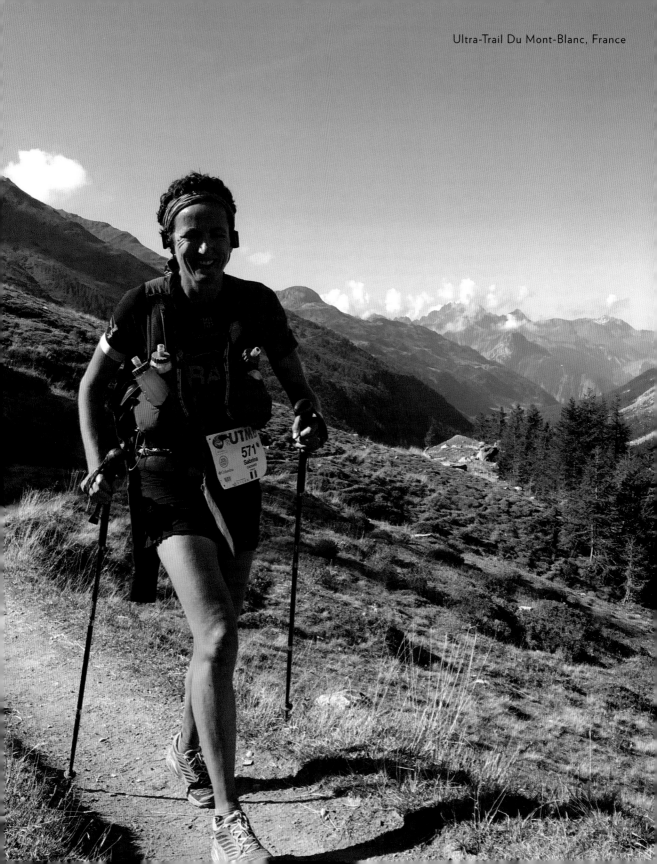

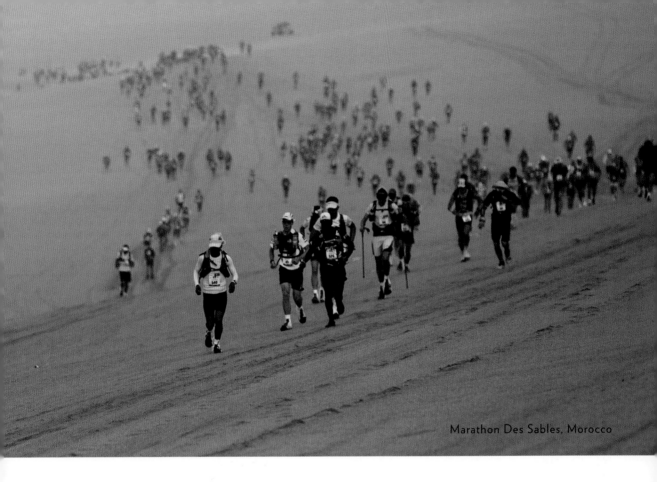

Marathon Des Sables, Morocco

MARATHON DES SABLES (MDS), MOROCCO

One of the world's most famous off-road races, billed 'The Toughest Footrace on Earth' but also very doable for many determined people who train hard and grit their teeth over seven days to cover 156 miles (250km) across endless sand dunes, blisteringly hot salt plains and rocky Saharan jebels (hills). This Moroccan epic was created in 1984 by French concert promoter Patrick Bauer, who went for a 200-mile (320km) walk in the desert with everything he needed on his back. He decided to create a similar experience for others, running the first event two years later with 186 competitors. It now attracts more than 1000 runners, including local legend Lahcen Ahansal, who has won it 10 times.

BARKLEY MARATHONS, USA

I'd hesitate to call this a trail race, but everyone needs to know about the ultimate kooky, crazy off-road event and its eccentric inventor! The race is based on a prison escape story, with an outrageously tough 60 miles (96.6km) over five loops through the impenetrable, bramble-choked forest around Frozen Head State Park in Tennessee. It's the brainchild of Lazarus Lake, who founded it in 1986 after hearing about Martin Luther King's escaped assassin only covering a tiny 8 miles (12.9km) in these woods from Brushy Mountain State Penitentiary after 55 hours in 1977. He thought he could have run further, so the Barkley Marathons was born. The race can start at any time Laz chooses from midnight to noon on race day. He blows a conch shell to signal the race will start in an hour's time, and it officially starts when he lights a cigarette. Most years, no one finishes, and the person Laz thinks is least likely to even complete one lap is given bib number 1 and called the 'human sacrifice'.

BOB GRAHAM ROUND, UK

This is fell running rather than trail running, and a challenge you take on whenever you like rather than an organised race, but it's very possibly Britain's most famous mountain run since Kilian Jornet broke Billy Bland's 36-year-old record on this 42-summit round in 2018. It's 65 miles (105km) in the Lake District, and the ascent of more than 8000m (26,247ft) across steep, rough ground, bog, rocks and scree makes it one of the hardest, most sought-after and well-respected badges of resilience and fitness in the off-road running world.

LAKELAND 50 AND 100, UK

This 50- or 100-mile (80km or 160km) trail race through the Lake District sells out almost immediately and is one of the UK's most popular ultras. The races have 3100m (10,170ft) and 6300m (20,670ft) of ascent respectively and the 100 weaves its way from the picturesque stone town of Coniston through green valleys, over mountain passes and beside stunning blue lakes. Half of the 100-milers fail to finish this course, but most of them get to the 50-mile (80km) point – where they probably wish they'd just signed up to the half-distance race! The shorter route also makes a good first 50-miler with its generous time limit of 24 hours, making it suitable for walkers as well as runners.

DRAGON'S BACK RACE, UK

A five-day epic across the entire mountainous spine of Wales, totalling almost 200 miles (320km) with more than 15,000m (49,210ft) of ascent. Billed as the 'toughest mountain race', it's not for the faint-hearted as you cross the notorious knife-edge scrambling ridge of Crib Goch and tackle steep, rock-choked and pathless terrain. First run in 1992 and won by a mixed pair, Helene Whitaker (née Diamantides) and Martin Stone, the race was reborn in 2012 and is now an annual event, drawing an international field.

TOR DES GÉANTS, ITALY

Italy's most celebrated race is a non-stop 205-mile (330km) ultra trail around the Italian Alps in the breathtakingly pointy Gran Paradiso National Park and the Aosta Valley. Runners tackle 25 mountain passes as they run in the shadow of the giants – Monte Cervino, Monte Rosa, Gran Paradiso and Monte Bianco. The total ascent is three times the height of Everest at 24,000m (78,740ft) and some years only 40 per cent of the runners finish the course, despite there being more than 2000 competitors from 76 countries.

YUKON ARCTIC ULTRA, CANADA

Following the Yukon Quest trail, competitors pull their sleds 100, 300 or 430 miles (160km, 480km or 700km) through the icy white snow in dangerously cold conditions. Known as the 'toughest ultra race in the world', the organisers warn that this event is genuinely life-threatening and you must sign a waiver to enter, but on the plus side you do get a free meal and hot water at every checkpoint.

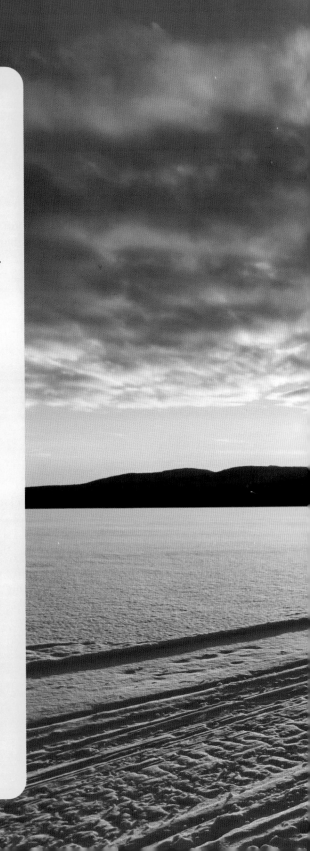

WORLD'S CRAZIEST RACES
Welcome to the less serious side of trail running with super-fun and unusual off-road events worldwide.

MAN V HORSE
Created by local Welsh blokes in a pub, only two men have beaten the horses over this rough, hilly and wet 22-mile (35km) course since the race was first run in 1982 from Llanwrtyd Wells in mid-Wales.

RACE THE TRAIN
Also in Wales, you can try to beat the train while your family cheer you on from the comfort of its carriages in a 14-mile (22.5km) run alongside the Talyllyn Railway from Abergynolwyn in south Snowdonia.

WIFE CARRYING
Originally from Finland, known as eukonkanto, these worldwide races originate from the terrifying tale of thieves who stole women away on their backs to marry, but it's now an amusing contest where the winner wins the weight of their 'wife' in beer.

HOBBY HORSE RACING
Again from Finland (what is it with the Finns and the Welsh?), young girls race and jump around a track with a hobby horse between their legs. Sounds fun! And a lot cheaper than actual horse riding...

BEER MILES
Held across the world, including at Love Trails Festival on the Gower Peninsula (South Wales), relay teams and solo competitors down a can of beer before sprinting a mile, preferably without vomiting – that would be cheating.

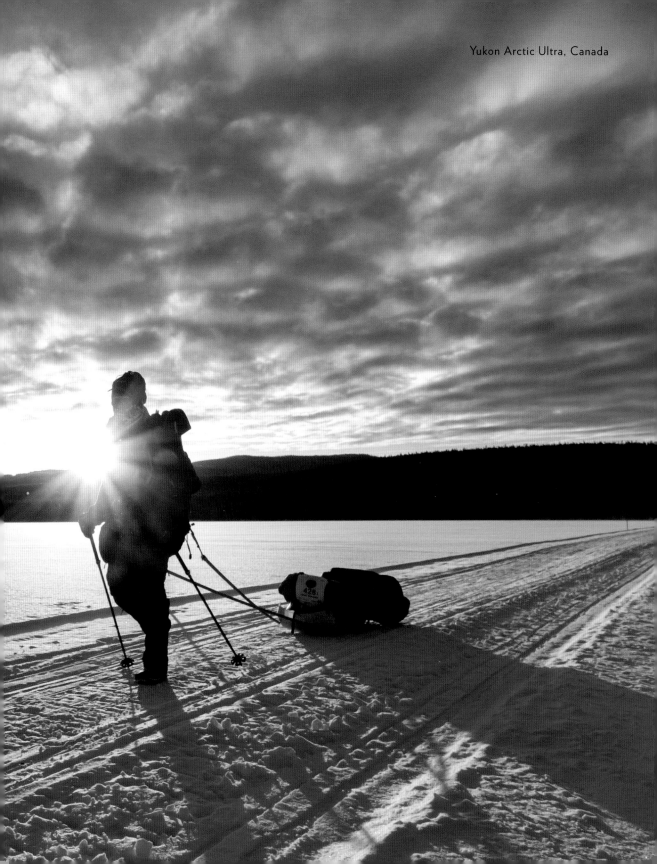

Yukon Arctic Ultra, Canada

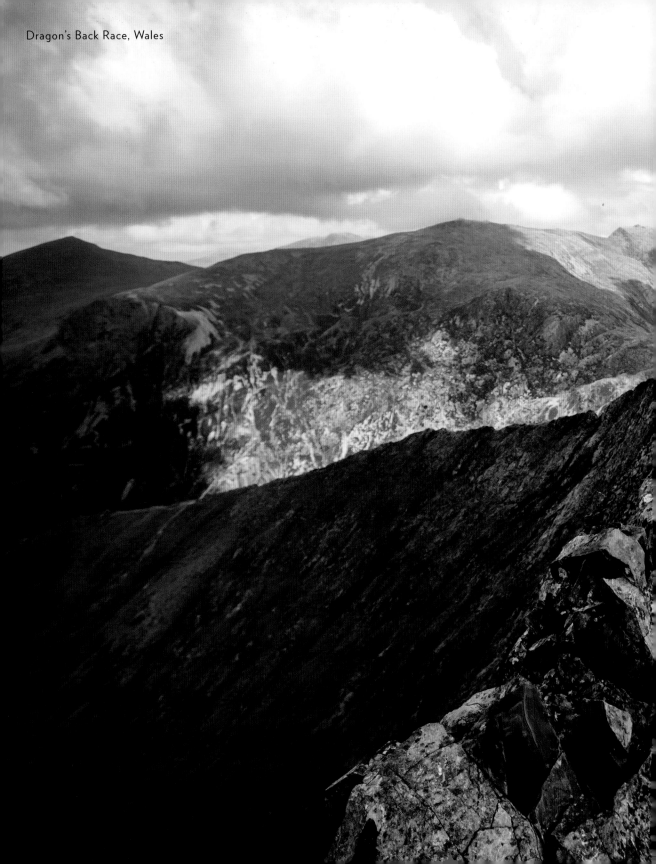

Dragon's Back Race, Wales

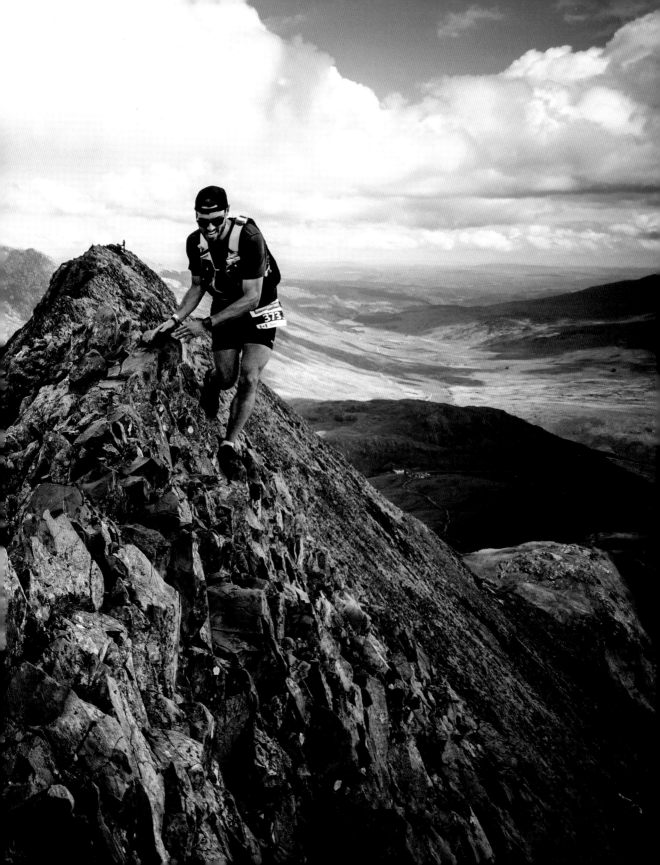

FURTHER READING

Now you've read this one, it's time for your next trail running book! Here are my all-time favourite off-road running reads.

Vassos Alexander, *Don't Stop Me Now* (Bloomsbury Sport, 2016)
A celebration of endurance running by popular sports presenter Vassos, who finds himself hooked on the infamous Dragon's Back Race and 153-mile Spartathlon, with chats with the world's most talented ultra runners along the way.

Richard Askwith, *Feet in the Clouds* (Aurum Press, 2013)
Warning: this book may inspire you to take on the ultimate fell running challenge, the Lake District's 65-mile (105km), 42-summit Bob Graham Round! This is journalist Richard's journey into fell running, which includes an engaging history of the sport.

Anita Bean, *The Runner's Cookbook* (Bloomsbury Sport, 2017)
More than 100 tasty, healthy recipes designed to fuel runners to peak performance and recovery, plus advice on all aspects of diet and fuelling from 5k to ultra, supplements and common mistakes, from qualified sports nutritionist Anita.

Steve Birkinshaw, *There is No Map in Hell* (Vertebrate Publishing, 2017)
A hugely eye-opening biography from one of Britain's most-loved endurance athletes. Steve overcame childhood setbacks to become a top orienteer, adventure racer and break Joss Naylor's 28-year-old record of 214 Wainwright summits.

Steve Chilton, *It's a Hill, Get Over It* (Sandstone Press Ltd, 2014)
A must-read for anyone interested in the history of British mountain, off-road and fell running (before trail running was invented!). Steve's book is an extremely well-researched and detailed encyclopedia for the sport.

Emelie Forsberg, *Sky Runner* (Hardie Grant Books, 2019)
A wonderful insight into the hard training and much-loved character of one of the world's best trail runners, with Emelie's own strength workouts, inspirational advice, delicious recipes and yoga moves.

**Damian Hall, *A Year on the Run*
(Aurum Press, 2016)**
A beautifully illustrated, very entertaining set of running stories to inspire you through 365 days of running by hill walker turned ultra runner Damian, who came fifth at the world-class Ultra-Trail du Mont-Blanc in 2018.

**Paul Hobrough, *Running Free of Injuries*
(Bloomsbury Sport, 2016)**
The best advice and exercises for preventing and rehabbing the most common running injuries, from foot to lower back, from Paul – physio to world-class, record-breaking runners Steve Cram and Paula Radcliffe.

**Kilian Jornet, *Run or Die*
(Viking, 2014)**
A fantastic way to get a good understanding of what makes the world's top trail runner tick, with stories that take you close to the bone. Kilian's first book is inspiring, scary and fascinating in equal measure.

**Scott Jurek, *Eat and Run*
(Bloomsbury Paperbacks, 2013)**
A fascinating insight into one of North America's best endurance athletes, his journey into ultra running, becoming veggie then vegan for performance, and running with the Tarahumara, plus all his favourite recipes.

**Christopher McDougall, *Born to Run*
(Profile Books, 2010)**
The original trail running book that inspired so many to run barefoot or in minimalist shoes. A hugely engaging account of top American ultra runners racing Mexico's elusive Tarahumara tribe of world-class runners.

**Anna McNuff, *The Pants of Perspective*
(Rocket 88, 2017)**
A hugely entertaining account of Anna's 148-day, 3000km (1864-mile) run from north to south New Zealand along the wild Te Araroa Trail, wearing her brightest running tights and learning about the power of resilience and self-belief.

ACKNOWLEDGEMENTS

I'd like to thank my always amazing hubby Steve and my whole family for the support, Mum and Jeanette for proofreading and helpful insights. Louise Lee, Hilary Cox, Katie Arnold, Francis Carlin, Janine Buck, Ed Fancourt and Julie Parker from Stamford Striders running club for the same.

Emelie Forsberg and Vassos Alexander for the great forewords.

Paul Hobrough for fab injury expertise.

Anita Bean for delicious nutrition expertise.

Shane Benzie for ace technique expertise.

Dave Taylor and Tim Pigott for wise words on the training plans.

Kirsty Reade for reading and advising.

The off-road athletes who shared their tips, the trail experts for their advice and the runners who shared their stories.

All my awesome Patreons, without whose support I could not do this.

PICTURE CREDITS

p. 7 (left) © Keswick Mountain Festival

pp. 18, 19 © www.inov-8.com;

p. 28 © Sam Greenhalgh;

pp. 21 (right), 22, 23, 26, 31, 41, 53, 54, 57, 61–65, 67–73, 77, 124–129, 134, 135, 136, 139, 140, 142–148, 152–159, 161, 163 (left), 165 (bottom), 167, 206, 207 by Andy Vernum Photography;

pp. 130–131 © Trail Running/H Bauer Publishing;

pp. 179 (right), 181 (right), 183 (right), 185 (right), 188, 192 by Adrian Lawrence Photography;

p. 214 © Mark Kelly and Montane, MYAU 2019;

pp. 216–217 © Dragon's Back Race® | No Limits Photography;

pp. 7 (right), 8, 10–11, 12, 20, 29, 123, 200, 203, 205, 211 © Claire Maxted;

pp. 5, 13, 14, 15, 17, 24, 25, 27, 30, 34, 35, 36–37, 38, 39, 40, 42, 44, 45, 47, 49, 50, 52, 56, 58–59, 60, 66, 74, 78, 80, 81, 82, 83, 95, 103, 111, 112–113, 114, 116, 117, 118, 119, 120, 121, 132–133, 141, 150, 151, 160, 163 (right), 165 (top), 168–169, 170, 172, 174, 175, 176, 178, 179 (left), 180, 181 (left), 182, 183 (left), 184, 185 (left), 186, 187, 189, 190, 193, 195, 196, 197, 198–199, 208, 212 © Getty Images

INDEX